D1558294

An Atlas of
ALZHEIMER'S DISEASE

THE ENCYCLOPEDIA OF VISUAL MEDICINE SERIES

An Atlas of
ALZHEIMER'S DISEASE

Edited by

Mony J. de Leon

Professor of Psychiatry and Director, Neuroimaging Laboratory
New York University School of Medicine and Nathan Kline Institute
New York, NY, USA

With contributions from

Heiko Braak, Khalid Iqbal, William J. Jagust
Judes Poirier, Barry Reisberg, Jerzy Wegiel
and Thomas Wisniewski

The Parthenon Publishing Group
International Publishers in Medicine, Science & Technology

NEW YORK   LONDON

Library of Congress Cataloging-in-Publication Data

An atlas of Alzheimer's disease / edited by Mony J. de Leon
      p. cm. -- (The encyclopedia of visual medicine series)
  Includes bibliographical references and index.
  ISBN 1-85070-912-2
  1. Alzheimer's disease Atlases. I. de Leon, Mony J. II. Series.
  [DNLM: 1. Alzheimer's Disease Atlases. WT 17 A881 1999]
RC523.A86 1999
616.8'31'022--dc21
DNLM/DLC
for Library of Congress   99-32886
                                                  CIP

British Library Cataloguing in Publication Data

An atlas of Alzheimer's disease. - (The encyclopedia of
  visual medicine series)
  1. Alzheimer's disease
  I. de Leon, Mony J.
  616.8'31

  ISBN 1-85070-912-2

Published in the USA by
The Parthenon Publishing Group Inc.
One Blue Hill Plaza
PO Box 1564, Pearl River
New York 10965, USA

Published in the UK and Europe by
The Parthenon Publishing Group Limited
Casterton Hall, Carnforth
Lancs. LA6 2LA, UK

Copyright ©1999 Parthenon Publishing Group
Illustrations featured in Chapter 2 Copyright
© 1999 by Barry Reisberg, M.D.

No part of this book may be reproduced in any form
without permission from the publishers, except for the
quotation of brief passages for the purposes of review.

Printed and bound in Spain by
T.G. Hostench, S.A.

Contents

List of contributors

Maciek Bobinski
Neuroimaging Laboratory
Department of Psychiatry
New York University School of Medicine
New York, NY, USA
and
Department of Pathological Neurobiology
New York State Institute for Basic Research in
  Developmental Disabilities
Staten Island, NY, USA

Eva Braak
Department of Anatomy
JW Goethe University
Frankfurt/Main, Germany

Heiko Braak
Department of Anatomy
JW Goethe University
Frankfurt/Main, Germany

Antonio Convit
Neuroimaging Laboratory
Department of Psychiatry
New York University School of Medicine
New York, NY, USA
and
Nathan Kline Institute
Orangeburg, NY, USA

Marc Danik
The McGill Centre for Studies in Aging
Douglas Hospital
Verdun, Quebec, Canada

Doris Dea
The McGill Centre for Studies in Aging
Douglas Hospital
Verdun, Quebec, Canada

Mony J. de Leon
Neuroimaging Laboratory
Department of Psychiatry
New York University School of Medicine
New York, NY, USA
and
Nathan Kline Institute
Orangeburg, NY, USA

Susan DeSanti
Neuroimaging Laboratory
Department of Psychiatry
New York University School of Medicine
New York, NY, USA

Blas Frangione
Department of Pathology
New York University Medical Center
New York, NY, USA

Emile H. Franssen
Aging and Dementia Research Center
Department of Psychiatry
New York University School of Medicine
New York, NY, USA

Inge Grundke-Iqbal
New York State Institute for Basic Research in
  Developmental Disabilities
Staten Island, NY, USA

Khalid Iqbal
New York State Institute for Basic Research in
  Developmental Disabilities
Staten Island, NY, USA

William J. Jagust
Department of Neurology
University of California Davis Medical Center
Sacramento, CA, USA

Judes Poirier
The McGill Centre for Studies in Aging
Douglas Hospital
Verdun, Quebec, Canada

Barry Reisberg
Aging and Dementia Research Center
Department of Psychiatry
New York University School of Medicine
New York, NY, USA

Chaim Tarshish
Neuroimaging Laboratory
Department of Psychiatry
New York University School of Medicine
New York, NY, USA

Jerzy Wegiel
Department of Pathological Neurobiology
New York State Institute for Basic Research in
  Developmental Disabilities
Staten Island, NY, USA

Henryk M. Wisniewski
Department of Pathological Neurobiology
New York State Institute for Basic Research in
  Developmental Disabilities
Staten Island, NY, USA

Thomas Wisniewski
Department of Neurology
New York University Medical Center
New York, NY, USA

1 Introduction and historical background
Mony J. de Leon

By the year 2030 it is estimated that between 17 and 20% or about 50 million of the population of the USA will be over age 65[1]. Dementia affects 1–6% of the population over the age of 65 and 10–20% over the age of 80[2], with its annual incidence approximately doubling for every 5 years of age between the ages of 75 and 89 years[3]. Other data currently show that, for every demented patient, there are many non-demented individuals with cognitive deterioration adversely affecting their quality of life[4]. Therefore, with respect to the above estimates, a staggering number of elderly with mild to severe cognitive impairments, perhaps 10–20 million, can be expected in the next 35 years, representing a great human and economic toll. Underlying the extensive research progress summarized in this text, is our shared hope that improved recognition of the risks for future Alzheimer's disease (AD), improved characterization of the natural history of AD, and the increased understanding of the neuropathy of AD will lead to early diagnosis, and to developing effective treatments. While the early diagnosis and the effective treatment of AD are topics of much interest today, our understandings are just beginning. The purpose of *An Atlas of Alzheimer's Disease* is to highlight the current clinical, anatomical and pathological knowledge bases that have shaped our understandings of AD. In putting together this text, the works from several leading research groups have been assembled. Collectively, these contributions offer a multidisciplinary view of the natural history of AD from its earliest brain manifestation to the globally debilitating end stage.

These assembled writings and illustrations converge to identify heuristically useful stages of disease progression across behavioral, neuroimaging, and neuropathology research areas. The Atlas also highlights and closely examines the major pathological brain lesions in AD and so provides an in-depth view of the neurofibrillary degeneration in AD and the beta-amyloid deposits in the brain. Finally, aspects of the new and rapidly unfolding genetic and molecular bases of the AD lesions are discussed.

We have targeted the materials presented in the Atlas to the student of Alzheimer's disease. We expect that this text will serve a wide base of readers as it provides both new and well-established information at several levels of difficulty and detail. Moreover, it presents some of the highest quality illustrations published to date in order to enhance communication of concepts and facts.

To further serve the interest of developing scholarship in the areas of human neurodegenerative diseases and brain aging, all the contributors have elected to donate their royalties from the sales of this text to a fund financing a young investigator research award. Moreover, David Bloomer, the President of The Parthenon Publishing Group, has generously agreed to double the royalty paid on all normal bookshop sales in order to substantially increase the prize fund available. We hope that this tradition will continue in future editions of the Atlas.

Finally, I wish to acknowledge the thousands of patients, their families and the normal volunteers who have participated in the studies reflected in the Atlas. These individuals have served others with the ultimate contributions – their time and their bodies.

2 Clinical stages of Alzheimer's disease

Barry Reisberg and Emile H. Franssen

Alzheimer's disease (AD) is a characteristic process with readily identifiable clinical stages. These clinical stages exist in a continuum with normal aging processes. The clinical stages of AD can be described in alternative ways. For example, they can be described globally or they can be described in terms of constituent elements, referred to as clinical axes. One of these clinical axes, functioning and self-care, is particularly useful in describing the progression of AD. However, many conditions, particularly in aged persons, can interfere with functioning apart from AD. For these and other reasons, functioning changes alone do not adequately describe the progress of AD. However, the combination of global changes and their functional concomitants can provide a clear map of the progress of AD. This clinical map is enriched by noting the common behavioral concomitants of the stages. However, the behavioral and mood manifestations of AD are much more diverse than the cognitive and functional features of the disease progression.

Globally, seven major stages from normality to most severe AD are identifiable[1,2]. Functionally, 16 stages and substages corresponding to the global stages are recognizable[3]. These global and functional clinical stages and substages of aging and AD are summarized as follows.

Stage 1: Normal

At any age, persons may potentially be free of objective or subjective symptoms of cognition and func-

tional decline and also free of associated behavioral and mood changes. We call these mentally healthy persons at any age, stage 1, or normal (Figure 1).

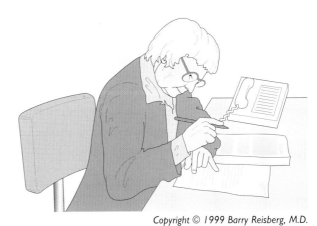

Figure 1 Stage 1: Normal

Stage 2: Normal aged forgetfulness

Half or more of the population of persons over the age of 65 experience subjective complaints of cognitive and/or functional difficulties. The nature of these subjective complaints is characteristic. Elderly persons with these symptoms believe they can no longer recall names as well as they could 5 or 10 years previously. They also frequently develop the conviction that they can no longer recall where they have placed things as well as previously (Figure 2). Subjectively experienced difficulties in concentra-

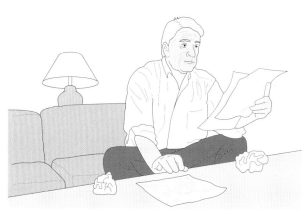

Figure 2 Stage 2: Normal aged subjective forgetfulness. 'Why can't I remember where I put those papers? I used to remember where everything that I put away was located'

tion and in finding the correct word when speaking, are also common. Various terms have been suggested for this condition, but normal aged forgetfulness is probably the most satisfactory terminology. These symptoms, which by definition, are not notable to intimates or other external observers of the person with normal aged forgetfulness, are generally benign[4]. However, there is some recent evidence that persons with these symptoms do decline at greater rates than similarly aged persons and similarly healthy persons who are free of subjective complaints[5].

Stage 3: Mild cognitive impairment

Persons at this stage manifest deficits which are subtle, but which are noted by persons who are closely associated with the stage 3 subject. The subtle deficits may become manifest in diverse ways. For example, the person with mild cognitive impairment (MCI) may noticeably repeat queries. The capacity to perform executive functions also becomes compromised. Commonly, for persons who are still working, job performance may decline. For those who must master new job skills, decrements in these capacities may become evident. For example, the MCI subject may be unable to master new computer skills (Figure 3). MCI subjects who are not employed, but who plan complex social

events, such as dinner parties, may manifest declines in their ability to organize such events. Other MCI subjects may manifest concentration deficits. Many persons with these symptoms begin to experience anxiety, which may be overtly evident[6].

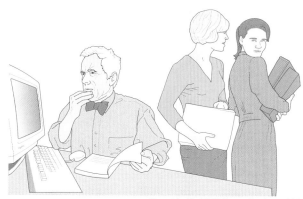

Figure 3 Stage 3: Mild memory impairment. In this stage, **ability to perform complex occupational and social tasks is compromised** and may be noticeable by colleagues. This is a 'border stage' which does not necessarily progress. When progression does occur, the true (potential) duration of this stage is probably 7 years; however, symptoms are commonly not observed until this stage has progressed at least midway through its temporal course

The prognosis for persons with these subtle symptoms of impairment is variable, even when a select subject group who are free of overt medical or psychological conditions which might account for, or contribute to, the impairments are studied. A substantial proportion of these persons will not decline, even when followed over the course of many years. However, in a majority of persons with stage 3 symptoms, overt decline will occur, and clear symptoms of dementia will become manifest over intervals of approximately 2 to 4 years[7]. In persons who are not called upon to perform complex occupational and/or social tasks, symptoms in this stage may not become evident to family members or friends of the MCI patient. Even when symptoms do become noticeable, MCI subjects are commonly midway or near the end of this stage before concerns result in clinical consultation. Consequently, although progression to the next stage in MCI subjects commonly occurs in 2 to 3 years, the true duration of this stage, when it is a harbinger of subsequently manifest dementia, is probably approximately 7 years[6].

Management of persons in this stage includes counseling regarding the desirability of continuing in a complex and demanding occupational role. Sometimes, a 'strategic withdrawal' in the form of retirement, may alleviate psychological stress and reduce both subjective and overtly manifest anxiety.

Stage 4: Mild Alzheimer's disease

Symptoms of impairment become evident in this stage. For example, seemingly major recent events, such as a recent holiday or a recent visit to a relative, may, or may not, be recalled. Similarly, overt mistakes in recalling the day of the week, month or season of the year may occur. Patients at this stage can still generally recall their correct current address. They can also generally correctly recall the weather conditions outside and very important current events, such as the name of a prominent head of state. Despite the overt deficits in cognition, persons at this stage can still potentially survive independently in community settings. However, functional capacities become compromised in the performance of instrumental (i.e. complex) activities of daily life. For example, there is a decreased capacity to manage personal finances. For the stage 4 patient who is living independently, this may become evident in the form of difficulties in paying rent and other bills. A spouse may note difficulties in writing the correct date and the correct amount in paying checks (Figure 4). The ability to independently market for food and groceries also becomes compromised in this stage. Persons who previously prepared meals for family members and/or guests begin to manifest decreased performance in these skills. Similarly, the ability to order food from a menu in a restaurant setting begins to be compromised. Frequently, this is manifest in the patient handing the menu to the spouse and saying 'you order'.

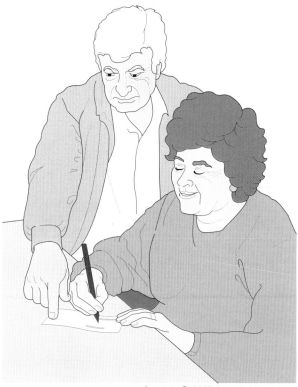

Figure 4 Stage 4: Mild Alzheimer's disease. The diagnosis of Alzheimer's disease can be made with considerable accuracy in this stage. The most common functioning deficit in these patients is a **decreased ability to manage instrumental (complex) activities of daily life**. Examples of common deficits include decreased ability to manage finances, to prepare meals for guests, and to market for oneself and one's family. The stage 4 patient shown has difficulty writing the correct date and the correct amount on the check. Consequently, her husband has to supervise this activity. The mean duration of this stage is 2 years

The dominant mood at this stage is frequently what psychiatrists term a flattening of affect and withdrawal. In other words, the patient often seems less emotionally responsive than previously. This absence of emotional responsivity is probably intimately related to the patient's denial of their deficit, which is often also notable at this stage. Although the patient is aware of their deficits, this awareness of decreased intellectual capacity is too painful for most persons and, hence, the psychological defense mechanism known as denial, whereby the patient seeks to hide their deficit, even from themselves where possible, becomes operative. In this context, the flattening of affect occurs because the patient is fearful of revealing their deficits. Consequently, the patient withdraws from participation in activities such as conversations.

In the absence of complicating medical pathology, the diagnosis of AD can be made with considerable certainty from the beginning of this stage. Studies indicate that the duration of this stage of mild AD is a mean of approximately 2 years.

Stage 5: Moderate Alzheimer's disease

At this stage, deficits are of sufficient magnitude as to prevent independent, catastrophe-free, community survival. Patients can no longer manage on their own in the community. If they are ostensibly alone in the community then there is generally someone who is assisting in providing adequate and proper food, as well as assuring that the rent and utilities are paid and the patient's finances are taken care of. For those who are not properly watched and/or supervised, predatory strangers may become a problem. Very common reactions for persons at this stage who are not given adequate support are behavioral problems such as anger and suspiciousness.

Cognitively, persons at this stage frequently cannot recall such major events and aspects of their current lives as the name of the current president, the weather conditions of the day, or their correct current address. Characteristically, some of these important aspects of current life are recalled, but not others. Also, the information is loosely held, so, for example, the patient may recall their correct address on certain occasions, but not others.

Remote memory also suffers to the extent that persons may not recall the names of some of the schools which they attended for many years, and from which they graduated. Orientation may be compromised to the extent that the correct year may not be recalled. Calculation deficits are of such magnitude

that an educated person has difficulty counting backward from 20 by 2s.

Functionally, persons at this stage have incipient difficulties with basic activities of daily life. The characteristic deficit of this type is decreased ability to independently choose proper clothing (Figure 5). This stage lasts an average of approximately 1.5 years[8].

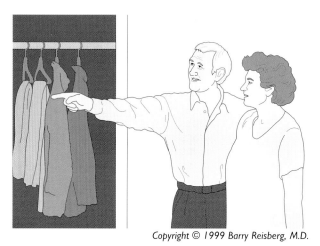

Copyright © 1999 Barry Reisberg, M.D.

Figure 5 Stage 5: Moderate Alzheimer's disease. In this stage, deficits are of sufficient magnitude as to prevent catastrophe-free, independent community survival. The characteristic functional change in this stage is **incipient deficits in basic activities of daily life**. This is manifest in a **decrement in the ability to choose proper clothing to wear** for the weather conditions and/or for the daily circumstances (occasions). Some patients begin to wear the same clothing day after day unless reminded to change. The spouse or other caregiver begins to counsel regarding the choice of clothing. The mean duration of this stage is 1.5 years

Stage 6: Moderately severe Alzheimer's disease

At this stage, the ability to perform basic activities of daily life becomes compromised. Functionally, five successive substages are identifiable. Initially, in stage 6a, patients, in addition to having lost the ability to choose their clothing without assistance, begin to require assistance in putting on their clothing properly. Unless supervised, patients may put their clothing on backward, they may have difficulty putting their arm in the correct sleeve, or they may

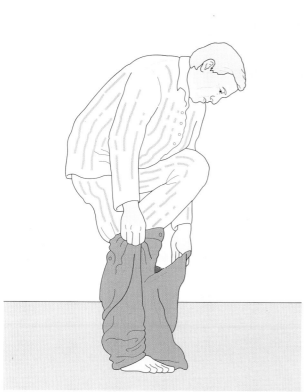

Figure 6 Stage 6a: Moderately severe Alzheimer's disease. In the stage of moderately severe Alzheimer's disease, the cognitive **deficits** are of sufficient magnitude as to **interfere with the ability to carry out basic activities of daily life**. Generally, the earliest such deficit noted in this stage is **decreased ability to put on clothing correctly without assistance**. The total duration of the stage of moderately severe AD (stage 6a through 6e) is approximately 2.5 years

dress themselves in the wrong sequence. For example, patients may put their street clothes on over their night clothes (Figure 6). At approximately the same point in the evolution of AD, but generally just a little later in the temporal sequence, patients lose the ability to bathe independently without assistance (stage 6b). Characteristically, the earliest and most common deficit in bathing is difficulty adjusting the temperature of the bath water (Figure 7). Initially, once the spouse adjusts the temperature of the bath water, the patient can still potentially otherwise bathe independently. Subsequently, as this stage evolves, additional deficits in bathing independently as well as in dressing independently

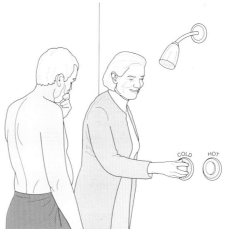

Figure 7 Stage 6b: Moderately severe Alzheimer's disease. Requires assistance adjusting the temperature of the bath water. At approximately the same time as Alzheimer's patients begin to lose the ability to put on their clothing properly without assistance, but generally just a little bit later in the disease course, patients begin to require assistance in handling the mechanics of bathing. Difficulty adjusting the temperature of the bath water is the classical earliest deficit in bathing capacity in Alzheimer's disease

occur. In this 6b substage, patients generally develop deficits in other modalities of daily hygiene such as properly brushing their teeth independently. With the further evolution of AD, patients lose the ability to manage independently the mechanics of toileting correctly (stage 6c). Unless supervised, patients may place the toilet tissue in the wrong place (Figure 8). Many patients will forget to flush the toilet properly. As the disease evolves in this stage, patients subsequently become incontinent. Generally, urinary incontinence occurs first (stage 6d), then fecal incontinence occurs (stage 6e). The incontinence can be treated, or even initially prevented entirely in many cases, by frequent toileting (Figure 9). Subsequently, strategies for managing incontinence, including appropriate bedding, absorbent undergarments, etc., become necessary.

In this sixth stage cognitive deficits are generally so severe that persons will display little or no knowledge when queried regarding such major aspects of their current life circumstances as their current address or the weather conditions of the day. Recall

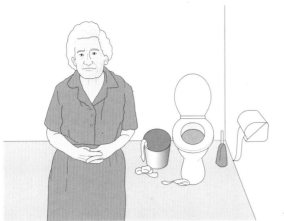

Figure 8 Stage 6c: Moderately severe Alzheimer's disease. **Requires assistance with cleanliness in toileting**. After Alzheimer's patients lose the ability to dress and bathe without assistance, they lose the ability to independently maintain cleanliness in toileting

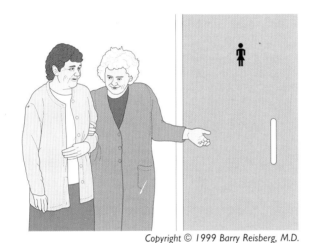

Figure 9 Stage 6d and 6e: Moderately severe Alzheimer's disease. **Requires assistance to maintain continence**. After Alzheimer's patients lose the ability to dress, bathe and toilet without assistance, they develop incontinence. Generally, urinary incontinence precedes fecal incontinence. Strategies to prevent episodes of incontinence include taking the patient to the restroom and supervision of toileting

of current events is generally deficient to the extent that the patient cannot name the current national head of state or other, similarly prominent newsworthy figures. Persons at this sixth stage will most often not be able to recall the names of any of the schools which they attended. They may, or may

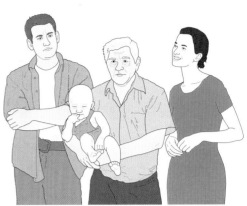

Figure 10 Stage 6: Moderately severe Alzheimer's disease. In this stage the patient's cognitive deficits are generally of such magnitude that the patient may at times confuse their wife with their mother or otherwise **misidentify or be uncertain of the identity of close family members**. At the end of this stage, speech ability overtly breaks down

not, recall such basic life events as the names of their parents, their former occupation and the country in which they were born. They still have some knowledge of their own names; however, patients in this stage begin to confuse their spouse with their deceased parent and otherwise mistake the identity of persons, even close family members, in their own environment (Figure 10). Calculation ability is frequently so severely compromised at this stage that even well-educated patients have difficulty counting backward consecutively from 10 by 1s.

Emotional changes generally become most overt and disturbing in this sixth stage of AD. Although these emotional changes may, in part, have a neurochemical basis, they are also clearly related to the patient's psychological reaction to their circumstances. For example, because of their cognitive deficits, patients can no longer channel their energies into productive activities. Consequently, unless appropriate direction is provided, patients begin to fidget, to pace, to move objects around and place items where they may not belong, or to manifest other forms of purposeless or inappropriate activities. Because of the patient's fear, frustration and shame regarding their circumstances, as well as other factors, patients frequently develop verbal outbursts, and threatening, or even violent, behavior may occur. Because patients can no longer survive independently, they commonly develop a fear of being left alone. Treatment of these and other behavioral and psychological symptoms which occur at this stage, as well as at other stages of AD, involves counseling regarding appropriate activities and the psychological impact of the illness upon the patient, as well as pharmacological interventions[9–12].

The mean duration of this sixth stage of AD is approximately 2.5 years[8]. As this stage comes to an end, the patient, who is doubly incontinent and needs assistance with dressing and bathing, begins to manifest overt breakdown in the ability to articulate speech. Stuttering (verbigeration), neologisms, and/or an increased paucity of speech, become manifest.

Stage 7: Severe Alzheimer's disease

At this stage, AD patients require continuous assistance with basic activities of daily life for survival. Six consecutive functional substages can be identified over the course of this final seventh stage. Early in this stage, speech has become so circumscribed, as to be limited to approximately a half dozen intelligible words or fewer in the course of an intensive contact and attempt at an interview with numerous queries (stage 7a). As this stage progresses, speech becomes even more limited to, at most, a single intelligible word (stage 7b). Once speech is lost, the ability to ambulate independently (without assistance), is invariably lost (stage 7c, Figure 11). However, ambulatory ability is readily compromised at the end of the sixth stage and in the early portion of the seventh stage by concomitant physical disability, poor care, medication side-effects or other factors. Conversely, superb care provided in the early seventh stage, and particularly in stage 7b, can postpone the onset of loss of ambulation, potentially for many years. However, under ordinary circumstances, stage 7a has a mean duration of approximately 1 year, and stage 7b has a mean duration of approximately 1.5 years[6,13]. In patients who remain alive, stage 7c lasts approximately 1 year[6,13], after which patients lose the ability not only to ambulate independently, but also to sit up inde-

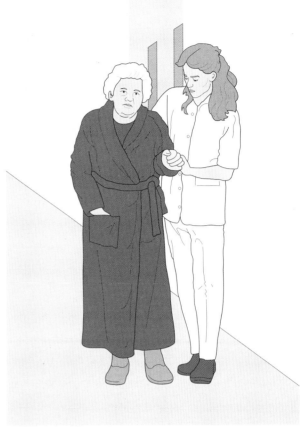

Figure 11 Stage 7: Severe Alzheimer's disease. Early in the course of this final stage of AD speech ability is limited to only a few words. Later, all intelligible speech is essentially lost, with speech limited to, at most, a single intelligible word. Subsequently, **ambulatory ability is lost and the patient requires assistance in walking**. Each substage of this final seventh stage lasts an average of 1–1.5 years

pendently (stage 7d). At this point in the evolution of AD, patients will fall over when seated unless there are arm rests to hold the patient up in the chair (Figure 12). This 7d substage lasts approximately 1 year[6,13]. Patients who survive subsequently lose the ability to smile (stage 7e). At this substage only grimacing facial movements are observed in place of smiles. This 7e substage lasts a mean of approximately 1.5 years[6,13]. It is followed in survivors, by a final 7f substage, in which AD patients additionally lose the ability to hold up their head independently.

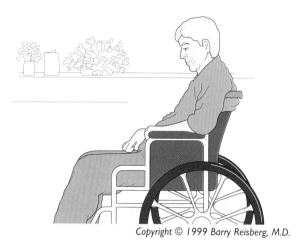

**Figure 12 Stage 7d: Severe Alzheimer's disease.
Without armrests on the chair, the patients
would fall over**. In the latter portion of the final stage
of AD, patients become immobile to the extent that they
require support to sit up without falling. With the
advance of this stage, patients lose the ability to smile
and, ultimately, to hold up their head without assistance,
unless their neck becomes contracted and immobile.
Patients can survive in this final 7f substage indefinitely;
however, most patients succumb during the course of
stage 7

With appropriate care and life support, patients can
survive in this final substage of AD for a period of
years.

With the advent of the seventh stage of AD, certain
physical and neurological changes become increasingly evident. One of these changes is physical
rigidity. Evident rigidity upon examination of the
passive range of motion of major joints, such as the
elbow, is present in the great majority of patients,
throughout the course of the seventh stage (Figure
13)[14,15]. In many patients, this rigidity appears to be
a precursor to the appearance of overt physical
deformities in the form of contractures.
Contractures are irreversible deformities which prevent the passive or active range of motion of joints
(Figure 14). In the early seventh stage (7a and 7b),
approximately 40% of AD patients manifest these
deformities[16]. Later in the seventh stage, in immobile patients (from stage 7d to 7f), nearly all AD
patients manifest contractures in multiple extremi-
ties and joints[16].

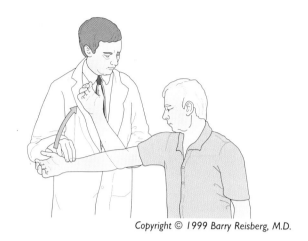

**Figure 13 In the final stages of AD patients mani-
fest increasing rigidity**. Rigidity is evident to the
examiner in the stage 7 patient upon passive range of
motion of major joints such as the elbow

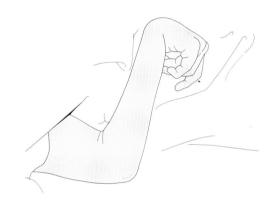

**Figure 14 Contractures of the elbow, wrists and
fingers**. Development of joint deformities known as
contractures, is an increasing problem in the stage 7
Alzheimer's disease. A contracture is a joint deformity
which makes full range of movement of a joint impossi-
ble without producing severe pain. Approximately 40%
of patients in stage 7a and 7b manifest these deformities
to the extent that they cannot move a major joint more
than half way. In the immobile Alzheimer's patient
(stages 7d to 7f), approximately 95% of patients manifest
these deformities which are usually present in many
joints

Neurological reflex changes also become evident in
the stage 7 AD patient. Particularly notable is the
emergence of so-called 'infantile', 'primitive' or
'developmental' reflexes which are present in the

infant but which disappear in the toddler. These reflexes, including the grasp reflex, sucking reflex (Figure 15), and the Babinski plantar extensor reflex (Figure 16), generally begin to re-emerge in the latter part of the sixth stage and are usually present in the stage 7 AD patient[17]. Because of the much greater physical size and strength of the AD patient in comparison with an infant, these reflexes can be very strong and can impact both positively and negatively on the care provided to the AD patient[18].

AD patients commonly die during the course of the seventh stage. The mean point of demise is when patients lose the ability to ambulate and to sit up

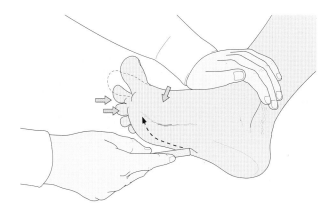

Copyright © 1999 Barry Reisberg, M.D.

Figure 16 Babinski or plantar extensor reflex. Another infantile reflex seen in the stage 7 Alzheimer's patient is the Babinski reflex. This abnormal response to stimulation of the sole of the foot is marked by dorsiflexion of the great toe and fanning of the other digits of the foot

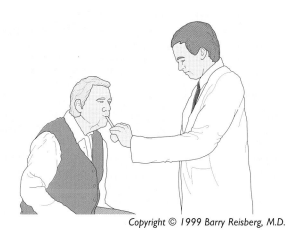

Copyright © 1999 Barry Reisberg, M.D.

Figure 15 Sucking reflex. 'Primitive' reflexes, also known as 'infantile' reflexes or 'developmental' reflexes, such as the sucking reflex, are evident in the stage 7 Alzheimer's patient

independently (stages 7c and 7d). The most frequent proximate cause of death is pneumonia. Aspiration is one common cause of terminal pneumonia. Another common cause of demise in AD is infected decubital ulcerations. AD patients in the seventh stage appear to be more vulnerable to all of the common causes of mortality in the elderly including stroke, heart disease and cancer. Some patients in this final stage appear to succumb to no identifiable condition other than AD.

Illustrations featured in Chapter 2
Copyright © 1999 by Barry Reisberg, M.D.

References

1. Reisberg B, Ferris SH, de Leon MJ, Crook T. The global deterioration scale for assessment of primary degenerative dementia. *Am J Psychiatry* 1982;139: 1136–9

2. Reisberg B, Sclan SG, Franssen EH, *et al.* Clinical stages of normal aging and Alzheimer's disease: the GDS staging system. *Neurosci Res Commun* 1993;13 (Suppl 1):551–4

3. Reisberg B. Functional assessment staging (FAST). *Psychopharmacol Bull* 1988;24:653–9

4. Flicker C, Ferris SH, Reisberg B. A longitudinal study of cognitive function in elderly persons with subjective memory complaints. *J Am Geriatr Soc* 1993; 41:1029–32

5. Geerlings MI, Jonker C, Bouter LM, *et al.* Association between memory complaints and incident Alzheimer's disease in elderly people with normal baseline cognition. *Am J Psychiatry* 1999;156:531–7

6. Reisberg B, Kluger A. Assessing the progression of dementia: diagnostic considerations. In Salzman C,

ed. *Clinical Geriatric Psychopharmacology*. Baltimore, 1998:432–62

7. Flicker C, Ferris SH, Reisberg B. Mild cognitive impairment in the elderly: predictors of dementia. *Neurology* 1991;41:1006–9

8. Reisberg B, Ferris SH, Franssen E, *et al*. Mortality and temporal course of probable Alzheimer's disease: a five-year prospective study. *Int Psychogeriatr* 1996,8:291–311

9. Reisberg B, Franssen E, Sclan SG, *et al*. Stage specific incidence of potentially remediable behavioral symptoms in aging and Alzheimer's disease: a study of 120 patients using the BEHAVE-AD. *Bull Clin Neurosci* 1989;54:95–112

10. Finkel SI, Costa e Silva JC, Cohen GD, *et al*. Behavioral and psychological symptoms of dementia: a consensus statement on current knowledge and implications for research and treatment. *Am J Geriatr Psychiatry* 1998;6:97–100

11. Reisberg B, Kenowsky S, Franssen EH, *et al*. President's Report: Towards a science of Alzheimer's disease management: a model based upon current knowledge of retrogenesis. *Int Psychogeriatr* 1999;11:7–23

12. Katz I, Jeste D, Mintzer JE, *et al*. Comparison of risperidone and placebo for psychosis and behavioral disturbances associated with dementia: a random-ized, double-blind trial. *J Clin Psychiatry* 1999; 60:107–15

13. Bobinski M, Wegiel J, Tarnawski M, *et al*. Relationships between regional neuronal loss and neurofibrillary changes in the hippocampal formation and duration and severity of Alzheimer disease. *J Neuropath Exp Neurol* 1997;56:414–20

14. Franssen EH, Reisberg B, Kluger A, *et al*. Cognition independent neurologic symptoms in normal aging and probable Alzheimer's disease. *Arch Neurol* 1991;48:148–54

15. Franssen EH, Kluger A, Torossian CL, Reisberg B. The neurologic syndrome of severe Alzheimer's disease. Relationship to functional decline. *Arch Neurol* 1993;50:1029–39

16. Souren LEM, Franssen EH, Reisberg B. Contractures and loss of function in patients with Alzheimer's disease. *J Am Geriatr Soc* 1995;43:650–5

17. Franssen EH, Souren LEM, Torossian CL, Reisberg B. Utility of developmental reflexes in the differential diagnosis and prognosis of incontinence in Alzheimer's disease. *J Geriatr Psychiatry Neurol* 1997;10:22–8

18. Souren LEM, Franssen EH, Reisberg B. Neuromotor changes in Alzheimer's disease: implications for patient care. *J Geriatr Psychiatry Neurol* 1997;10:93–8

3 Positron emission tomography and single-photon emission computed tomography in dementia

William J. Jagust

Traditional approaches to brain imaging in evaluating demented patients have emphasized the use of structural brain imaging to exclude reversible causes of dementia. This view is slowly undergoing re-examination, along with the general approach to the diagnosis of dementia as a diagnosis of exclusion. Over the past decade, reliable and valid diagnostic criteria for a number of different dementias have been promoted, especially for Alzheimer's disease (AD)[1]. These criteria have focused diagnostic approaches on 'ruling in' specific dementias rather than 'ruling out' treatable causes.

Along with this change in thinking comes increasing interest in diagnostic tests that support or confirm specific dementia diagnoses. In particular, functional brain imaging with techniques like positron emission tomography (PET) and single-photon emission computed tomography (SPECT) have been proposed to provide additional information about brain function that can assist in the clinical diagnosis of a variety of dementias.

AD is the dementing illness that had received the most attention in the neuroimaging literature, and a number of functional imaging markers have been suggested as being characteristic of the diagnosis. The primary markers include hypoperfusion in the temporal and parietal lobes on SPECT imaging, hypoperfusion and hypometabolism in temporoparietal cortex and posterior cingulate cortex in PET imaging[2-7]. These functional flow and metabolic deficits parallel the severity and nature of cognitive disturbances, are frequently asymmetric, and occur early in the disease[8-10]. There does not appear to be any difference in PET scan appearance based on genetic etiologies[11,12].

The specific diagnostic utility of these patterns remains disputed, partially because large-scale studies with heterogeneous samples and autopsy validation have not been performed. Nevertheless, SPECT perfusion imaging in AD patients in comparison to controls generally produces estimates of sensitivity and specificity of the order of 80–90%[13,14]. A number of dementias show metabolic and perfusion patterns that differ considerably from AD, particularly fronto-temporal dementias, including Pick's disease[15-17]. The pattern of frontal hypometabolism is not specific for this diagnosis, as it has been reported in progressive supranuclear palsy[18,19] and in some cases of vascular dementia[20]. In addition, patients with progressive syndromes of focal cortical degeneration, such as primary progressive aphasia, may show patterns quite distinct from AD[21,22]. Areas where imaging findings have been diagnostically confusing are vascular dementia and Parkinson's disease with dementia, both of which may show patterns similar to the pattern of temporoparietal hypometabolism seen in AD[23-25].

Although precise sensitivity, specificity, and diagnostic utility of these imaging markers are still debatable, the robust nature of many of the findings has prompted investigators to explore whether they are useful for identifying individuals who are

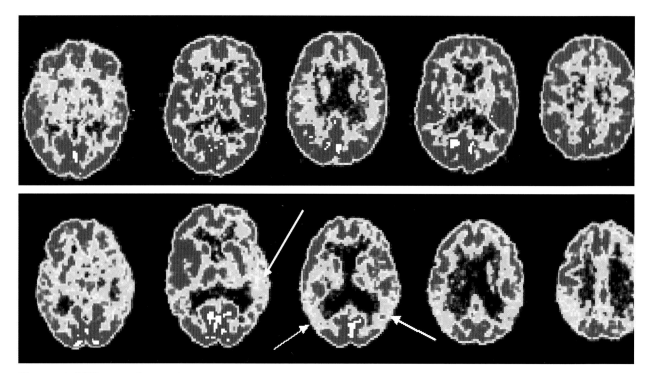

Figure I PET scans from a healthy older control subject (upper) and a patient with AD (lower), showing the regional cerebral metabolic rate for glucose (rCMRglc), using the metabolic tracer [^{18}F]-fluorodeoxyglucose (FDG). The level of glucose metabolism correlates with color intensity, with the higher colors (white, red) indicative of greater glucose metabolism.

The control subject shows a relatively even cortical distribution of FDG whereas the AD patient shows reduced glucose metabolism predominantly in the parietal cortex bilaterally (white arrows). This hypometabolism is relatively symmetrical in the parietal lobes although, more ventrally, the reduction in the temporal lobes (yellow arrow) is greater in the left hemisphere than in the right. Many studies have observed that metabolic asymmetry is correlated with behavioral deficit. Thus, this AD patient may have exhibited an aphasia as a predominant cognitive disturbance.

This difference in glucose metabolism in normal aging *vs* AD has been proposed as a useful diagnostic tool in the evaluation of dementia patients as healthy older subjects do not show the typical AD pattern. However, many questions remain concerning the true diagnostic utility of these appearances. The precise sensitivity and specificity in unselected, unbiased samples is not clear nor is there sufficient autopsy data to support differentiation of AD from other dementias. Nevertheless, small series have suggested that a number of other dementias differ from AD in their patterns of metabolic abnormalities

affected by AD but who have not yet expressed the disease.

Functional brain imaging has been used to evaluate those at risk of developing dementia in a number of studies. Small and colleagues[26] used PET and the fluorodeoxyglucose method and found that mildly impaired relatives of AD patients with the apolipoprotein e4 allele had lower parietal metabolism than clinically similar subjects without this risk factor. Kennedy and colleagues[27] found that a group

of at-risk subjects from families with autosomal dominant AD (chromosome 14 and 21 etiologies) had reduced global and temporoparietal glucose metabolism compared with a control group. Reiman and colleagues[28] studied a group of individuals with normal cognitive function who were homozygous for the e4 allele, and found reductions in temporal and parietal glucose metabolism, with greatest reductions in the posterior cingulate cortex. Taken together, these three studies clearly demonstrate abnormalities in association neocortex in individuals likely to develop AD. To date, there has been no demonstration of predictive ability in individual subjects. Using SPECT, Johnson and colleagues[29] found perfusion patterns in subjects with questionable dementia who progressed to clearcut AD different from those in subjects who did not progress. In this study, functional changes included medial temporal structures and cingulate gyrus.

In this chapter, brain images representative of the sorts of findings that may be clinically useful are presented. These images provide an overview of functional brain changes that occur in a number of different dementias, and that can provide information of clinical utility in ruling in a number of different etiologies of dementia.

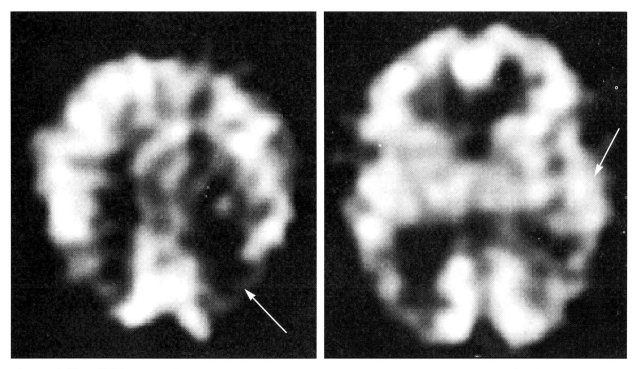

Figure 2 Two SPECT scans from a patient with AD using n-isopropyl-p-iodoamphetamine (IMP) as a tracer for regional cerebral blood flow (rCBF). In AD, rCBF parallels rCMRglc because of reduced demand. Thus, perfusion tracers used with a variety of techniques (SPECT, PET, MRI or collimated probes) demonstrate reduced perfusion in the same areas of the temporal and parietal cortices as are seen in FDG scans.

In this AD patient, blood flow reductions are seen at the level of the parietal lobes (left) and temporal lobes (right)

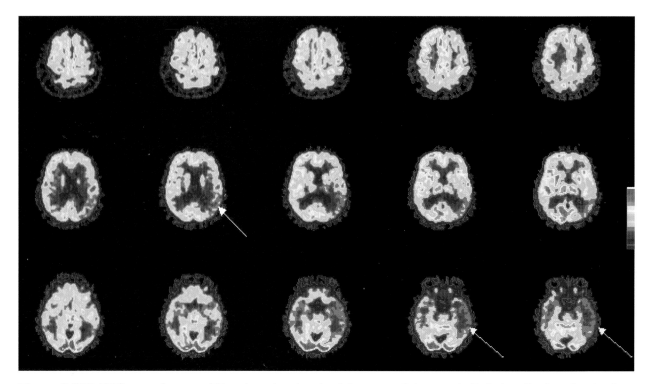

Figure 3 PET–FDG scans from an AD patient showing the full extent of the metabolic lesion. Profound reductions are seen throughout the temporal cortex (yellow arrows) and extend dorsally through the parietal cortex (white arrow). This metabolic decrement is asymmetrical, with greater abnormality in the left hemisphere.

Two other points are clearly demonstrated by this series of images. First, there is relative preervation of primary sensory and motor cortex. Bright (red) areas are evident in the somatosentory cortex bilaterally as well as in the primary visual cortex posteriorly. Basal ganglia are also preserved. In addition, the temporal lobe shows severe involvement in the lateral neocortical aspect whereas the mesial aspect is not as severely involved. Although it may appear reasonable to assume the presence of severe and invariable metabolic abnormality in the mesial temporal cortex, this is not invariably seen in AD patients

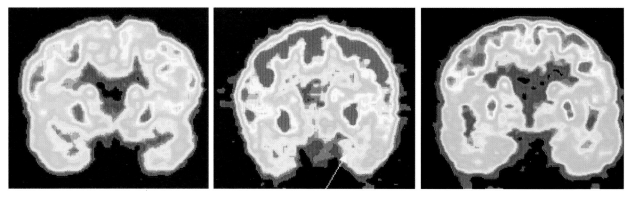

Figure 4 Coronal PET scans from two control subjects (left and right) and an AD patient (middle). This view is better for visualizing mesial temporal structures. The AD patient shows reduced rCMRglc in the mesial temporal lobes (yellow arrow) compared with the neocortex, which is consistent with the observation that, in some AD patients, mesial temporal lobe metabolism is indeed reduced. In contrast, the controls show markedly different metabolic patterns: one (right) demonstrates preserved mesial temporal lobe metabolism; the other (left) shows reductions in rCMRglc in the same region. These variations in mesial temporal metabolism with normal aging may be one of the factors contributing to the difficulties in using this metabolic finding as a marker for AD

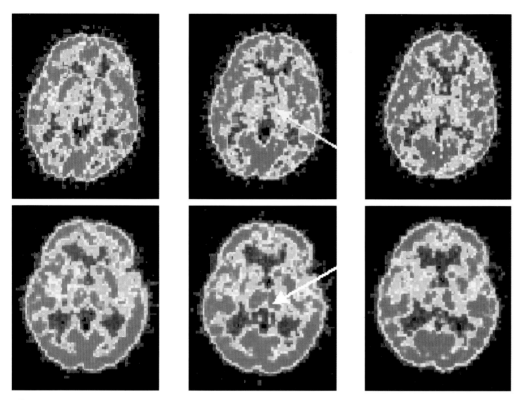

Figure 5 A number of other dementias show metabolic or perfusion patterns distinct from that of AD, as demonstrated in these PET–FDG scans from a patient with familial fatal insomnia (FFI; upper) compared with a control (lower). FFI patients are reported to have reduced rCMRglc in the thalamus, which parallels the distribution of prion protein, as seen in this FFI patient in whom metabolism in the thalamus is barely visible (arrowed). In contrast, the normal control shows relatively high levels of metabolism in the thalamus (arrowed)

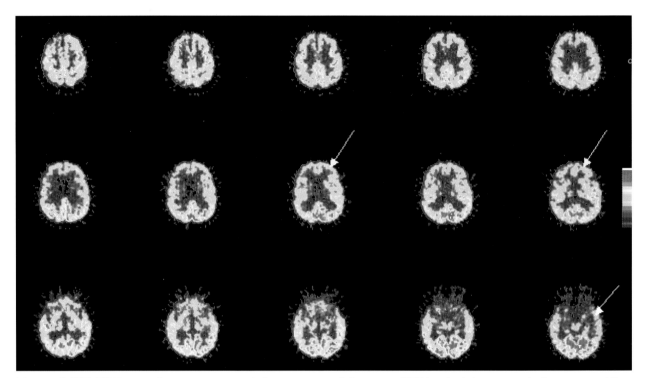

Figure 6 PET–FDG scans from a patient with frontotemporal dementia (FTD), which has a metabolic pattern different from that of AD. In this FTD patient, metabolic decrements are prominent in the frontal lobes (yellow arrows) as well as in both dorsolateral and orbitofrontal regions. In addition, there are reductions in the anterior temporal lobes (white arrow).

Patients with AD usually present with amnesia as the primary symptom. In contrast, FTD patients generally demonstrate profound behavioral disturbances and aphasias early in the disease, reflecting the relative involvement of the frontal and anterior temporal regions in these patients rather than the posterior temporal, parietal and mesial temporal regions involved in AD

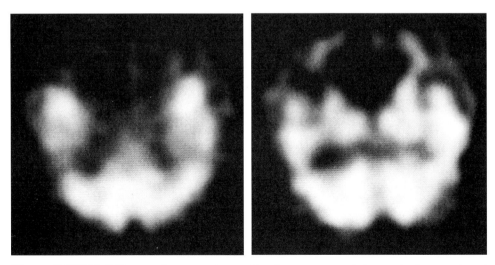

Figure 7 SPECT–IMP scans from a patient with a frontotemporal dementia show reduced perfusion in both dorsolateral frontal (left) and orbitofrontal (right) lobes. As seen in AD, reductions in perfusion appear to follow reductions in glucose metabolism, presumably because of reduced metabolic demand

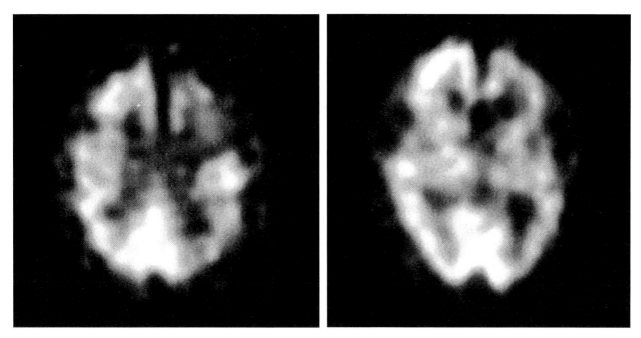

Figure 8 SPECT–IMP scans from a patient with primary progressive aphasia (PPA) syndrome. In this case, the hypometabolism is confined to the left hemisphere. Patients with PPA experience slowly progressive aphasias without concomitant dementia although, later in the disease, dementia may supervene. PPA has been associated with a number of pathological findings, including AD and FTD, together with less specific neuropathological changes. Functional brain imaging may help in the differential diagnosis as lateralized hypoperfusion or hypometabolism, which persists well into the course of the disease, is rarely the sole manifestation of either AD or FTD. The presence of either a bilateral temporoparietal or a bilateral frontal pattern of hypofunction is strong evidence that either AD or FTD is present

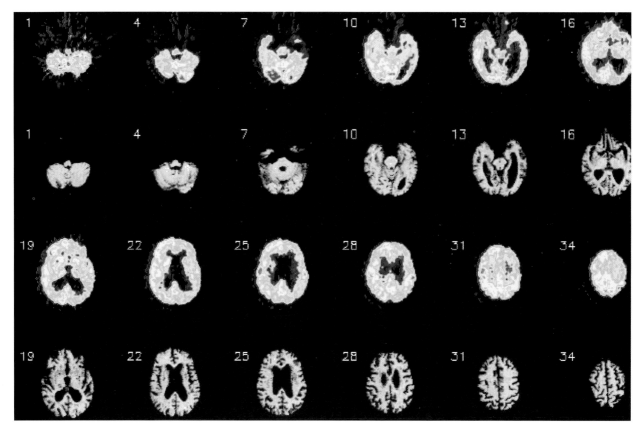

Figure 9 PET–FDG and MRI scans from a patient with ischemic vascular dementia who had multiple subcortical infarcts. The PET scans show hypometabolism lateralized to the left hemisphere. Thus, although this pattern is considered characteristic of PPA syndrome, it is seen in other conditions. In this patient, the laterality of the metabolic lesions parallels the laterality of the structural lesions. In fact, vascular dementia is not associated with a particular pattern of hypometabolism as the pattern is dependent upon the location of cerebral infarcts. Vascular dementia may mimic most patterns of hypometabolism, including that of AD or FTD, if lesions are located in appropriate places (temporoparietal cortex and connections, or frontal cortex and related subcortical circuitry)

References

1. McKhann G, Drachman D, Folstein M, *et al.* Clinical diagnosis of Alzheimer's disease: report of the NINCDS-ADRDA work group under the auspices of Department of Health and Human Services Task Force on Alzheimer's Disease. *Neurology* 1984;34:939–44

2. Frackowiak RSJ, Pozzili C, Legg NJ, *et al.* Regional cerebral oxygen supply and utilization in dementia: a clinical and physiological study with oxygen-15 and positron tomography. *Brain* 1981;104:753–78

3. Minoshima S, Giordani B, Berent S, *et al.* Metabolic reduction in the posterior cingulate cortex in very early Alzheimer's disease. *Ann Neurol* 1997;42:85–94

4. Ibáñez V, Pietrini P, Alexander GE, *et al.* Regional glucose metabolic abnormalities are not the result of atrophy in Alzheimer's disease. *Neurology* 1998;50:1585–93

5. Sharp P, Gemmell H, Cherryman G, *et al.* Application of iodine-123-labeled isopropylamphetamine imaging to the study of dementia. *J Nucl Med* 1986;27:761–8

6. Jagust WJ, Budinger TF, Reed BR. The diagnosis of dementia with single photon emission computed tomography. *Arch Neurol* 1987;44:258–62

7. Johnson KA, Mueller ST, Walshe TM, *et al.* Cerebral perfusion imaging in Alzheimer's disease: use of sin-

gle photon emission computed tomography and iofetamine hydrochloride I 123. *Arch Neurol* 1987;44: 165–8

8. Friedland RP, Budinger TF, Koss E, *et al.* Alzheimer's disease: anterior–posterior and lateral hemispheric alterations in cortical glucose utilization. *Neurosci Lett* 1985;53:235–40

9. Haxby JV, Duara R, Grady CL, *et al.* Relations between neuropsychological and cerebral metabolic asymmetries in early Alzheimer's disease. *J Cerebral Blood Flow Metab* 1985;5:193–200

10. Reed BR, Jagust WJ, Seab JP, *et al.* Memory and regional cerebral blood flow in mildly symptomatic Alzheimer's disease. *Neurology* 1989;39:1537–9

11. Kennedy AM, Rossor MN, Frackowiak RSJ. Positron emission tomography in familial Alzheimer's disease. *Alzheimer Dis Assoc Disord* 1995;9:17–20

12. Corder EH, Jelic V, Basun H, *et al.* No difference in cerebral glucose metabolism in patients with Alzheimer's disease and differing apolipoprotein E genotypes. *Arch Neurol* 1997;54:273–7

13. Johnson KA, Holman BL, Rosen TJ, *et al.* Iofetamine I 123 single photon emission computed tomography is accurate in the diagnosis of Alzheimer's disease. *Arch Intern Med* 1990;150:752–6

14. Eberling JL, Jagust WJ, Reed BR, *et al.* Reduced temporal lobe blood flow in Alzheimer's disease. *Neurobiol Aging* 1992;13:483–91

15. Jagust WJ, Reed BR, Seab JP, *et al.* Clinical-physiologic correlates of Alzheimer's disease and frontal lobe dementia. *Am J Physiol Imaging* 1989;4:89–96

16. Neary D, Snowden JS, Northen B, *et al.* Dementia of frontal lobe type. *J Neurol Neurosurg Psychiatr* 1988;51:353–61

17. Miller BL, Cummings JL, Villaneuva-Meyer J, *et al.* Frontal lobe degeneration: clinical neuropsychological, and SPECT characteristics. *Neurology* 1991;41:1374–82

18. D'Antona R, Baron JC, Samson Y, *et al.* Subcortical dementia: frontal cortex hypometabolism detected by positron emission tomography in patients with progressive supranuclear palsy. *Brain* 1985;108: 785–99

19. Foster NL, Gilman S, Berent S, *et al.* Cerebral hypometabolism in progressive supranuclear palsy studied with positron emission tomography. *Ann Neurol* 1988;24:399–406

20. Cohen MB, Graham LS, Lake R, *et al.* Diagnosis of Alzheimer's disease and multiple infarct dementia by tomographic imaging of iodine-123 IMP. *J Nucl Med* 1986;27:769–74

21. Chawluk JB, Mesulam M-M, Hurtig H, *et al.* Slowly progressive aphasia without generalized dementia: studies with positron emission tomography. *Ann Neurol* 1986;19:68–74

22. Caselli RJ, Jack CR, Petersen RC, *et al.* Asymmetric cortical degenerative syndromes: clinical and radiologic correlations. *Neurology* 1992;42:1462–8

23. Kuhl DE, Metter EJ, Riege WH. Patterns of local cerebral glucose utilization determined in Parkinson's disease by the [18F]Fluoro-deoxyglucose method. *Ann Neurol* 1984;15:419–24

24. Peppard RF, Martin WRW, Carr GD, *et al.* Cerebral glucose metabolism in Parkinson's disease with and without dementia. *Arch Neurol* 1992;49:1262–8

25. Eberling JL, Jagust WJ, Reed BR, *et al.* Single-photon emission computed tomography studies of regional cerebral blood flow in multiple infarct dementia. *J Neuroimag* 1992;2:79–85

26. Small GW, Mazziotta JC, Collins MT, *et al.* Apolipoprotein E type 4 allele and cerebral glucose metabolism in relatives at risk for familial Alzheimer's disease. *J Am Med Assoc* 1995;273:942–7

27. Kennedy AM, Frackowiak RSJ, Newman SK, *et al.* Deficits in cerebral glucose metabolism demonstrated by positron emission tomography in individuals at risk of familial Alzheimer's disease. *Neurosci Lett* 1995;186:17–20

28. Reiman EM, Caselli RJ, Yun LS, *et al.* Preclinical evidence of Alzheimer's disease in persons homozygous for the e4 allele for apolipoprotein E. *N Engl J Med* 1996;334:752–8

29. Johnson KA, Jones K, Holman BL, *et al.* Preclinical prediction of Alzheimer's disease using SPECT. *Neurology* 1998;50:1563–71

4 MRI studies of the hippocampal formation: contributions to the early diagnosis of Alzheimer's disease

Mony J. de Leon, Antonio Convit, Chaim Tarshish, Susan DeSanti and Maciek Bobinski

Cross-sectional and longitudinal clinical studies commonly observe subtle declines in cognitive functioning associated with aging, and the underlying brain anatomy and physiological mechanisms responsible for these age-related declines in cognition are becoming better understood. Recent neuropathology and structural neuroimaging studies consistently point to the hippocampal formation as a key structure in understanding age-related cognitive changes, particularly memory impairments.

Recent neuropathology studies (see Chapter 5) identify the neurons of the hippocampal formation (see below) as most vulnerable to the age-related deposition of neurofibrillary tangles (NFT), a diagnostic feature of AD[5]. Moreover, for many elderly patients with mild cognitive impairments (MCI) (see Chapter 2), NFT deposition in the hippocampal formation is a relatively focal anatomical insult[6]. With progression of the clinical disease, there is a correlated progression of the neuropathology to include involvement of the neocortex[5]. *In vivo* neuroimaging studies have similarly demonstrated anatomically specific volume reductions in the hippocampus of MCI patients; with increasing clinical severity this specific alteration gives way to general neocortical volume losses[7].

As a group, MCI patients are at increased risk of developing symptoms of AD within a few years. Longitudinal neuroimaging studies show that both hippocampal volume and measures of delayed recall are accurate predictors of future dementia in MCI patients. In both neuropathology and neuroimaging studies, the dementia symptoms of AD are associated with hippocampal formation and neocortical pathology. These observations have led Braak and colleagues to the proposition that AD-related neuropathology follows over time a relatively orderly pattern that enables one to identify stages of involvement. Such a proposition now applies to structural neuroimaging. As we improve our ability to detect, *in vivo*, the anatomic changes in the hippocampal formation, so we increase our identification of patients at increased risk for adverse memory changes and ultimately AD.

The purpose of this chapter is threefold: first, to describe the normal anatomy of the hippocampal formation, and describe the anatomy vulnerable to neuropathological changes in both normal aging and AD. Particular emphasis will be placed on the anatomy visible with *in vivo* structural neuroimaging; second, to review relationships between hippocampal formation damage and neuropsychological performances; and, third, to review the data in support of the hypothesis that hippocampal formation atrophy occurs early in the natural history of AD and precedes neocortical involvement.

Hippocampal formation neuroanatomy

The hippocampal formation is one of the major parts of the allocortex (a phylogenetically older cortex that is part of the rhinencephalon). It comprises the hippocampus proper (hippocampus), dentate gyrus, subicular complex and the entorhinal cortex[8,9].

General boundaries of the hippocampus

The hippocampus, a temporal lobe structure, is particularly well developed in the human brain. It is located on the floor of the temporal (inferior) horn of the lateral ventricle. The hippocampus is known for its seahorse-like appearance and much of its gross anatomy can be viewed with magnetic resonance imaging (MRI). The length of the hippocampus is about 4–5 cm, with a maximal width of about 2 cm and a maximal height of about 1.5 cm[10].

The boundaries of the hippocampus vary along its rostrocaudal length. To illustrate these boundaries at four levels along the hippocampal length, we utilize both *in vivo* T_1 weighted MRI scans and postmortem sections stained with creysl violet (Figure 1). Note that the numbers in brackets in the text correspond to those indicated in the figure. Figures 1a and b represent the anterior hippocampus at the level of the amygdaloid body. At this level, the hippocampus [1] is bounded dorsally by the amygdala [2], laterally by the temporal horn [3], inferiorly by the subiculum [4] and the white matter of the parahippocampal gyrus [5], and medially by the ambient cistern [6]. The anterior parahippocampal gyrus [5] is bounded laterally by the collateral sulcus [7], and contains the entorhinal [8] and transentorhinal cortices as its inferior boundary. At the amygdala level, the entorhinal cortex extends medially to cover the ambiens [9] and semilunar [10] gyri. Although the boundary between the hippocampus and the amygdala is somewhat indistinct, the visual separation between amygdala and hippocampus can be facilitated using sagittal views, which are readily obtained with MRI[11]. More posteriorly, at the level of the hippocampal head (also referred to as pes hippocampus or uncus) (Figures 1c and d), the hippocampus [1] is more complex in shape. The temporal horn [3] is found laterally. Inferiorly are found the uncal sulcus [11], the white matter of the parahippocampal gyrus and the subiculum [4]; superiorly the choroid plexus of the temporal horn [3a]; and medially the ambient cis-

tern [6]. The parahippocampal gyrus is bounded inferiorly and medially by the tentorium cerebelli [12] and laterally by the collateral sulcus. The entorhinal cortex, a part of the parahippocampal gyrus (see below), is generally found at the pes hippocampal level and is mainly bounded between the lateral collateral sulcus and the medial aspect (uncus) of the parahippocampal gyrus. Posterior levels of the pes hippocampus have the shape of a figure of eight lying on its side.

Figures 1e and f represent the level of the body of the hippocampus. At this level, the lateral and superior hippocampus boundaries are the temporal horn [3] and choroid plexus of the lateral ventricle. The inferior boundary is the subiculum [4] and the white matter of the parahippocampal gyrus [5]. On the dorsal and medial border of the hippocampus is the fimbria [13], which is made up of white matter fibers that extend posteriorly to form the fornix. The cerebrospinal fluid (CSF) space medial to the body of the hippocampus is the transverse fissure of Bichat [14], which medially separates the subiculum [4] from the thalamus [15] (see lateral geniculate level figure) over the length of the body and tail of the hippocampus.

Figures 1g and h represent the tail of the hippocampus at the level of the splenium of the corpus callosum [17]. At this level, the hippocampus [1] is inferior and lateral to the fornix [16] and the splenium of the corpus callosum.

The hippocampus

The individual fields of the hippocampus can be pictured as a stacked bundle of tissue strips running rostrocaudally in the temporal lobe. The distinctive C-shape of the hippocampus is present when the bundled strips fold over each other mediolaterally as seen in the midportion or body of the hippocampus (see Figure 1f). On more rostral sections, the hippocampus bends sharply in a medial and then in a caudal direction. The more rostral levels of the hippocampal structure are more complex, mostly owing to a varied number of rostrocaudal flexures. At caudal levels (hippocampal tail), the hippocampus bends dorsally and ascends towards the splenium. As a part of the allocortex, the cornu

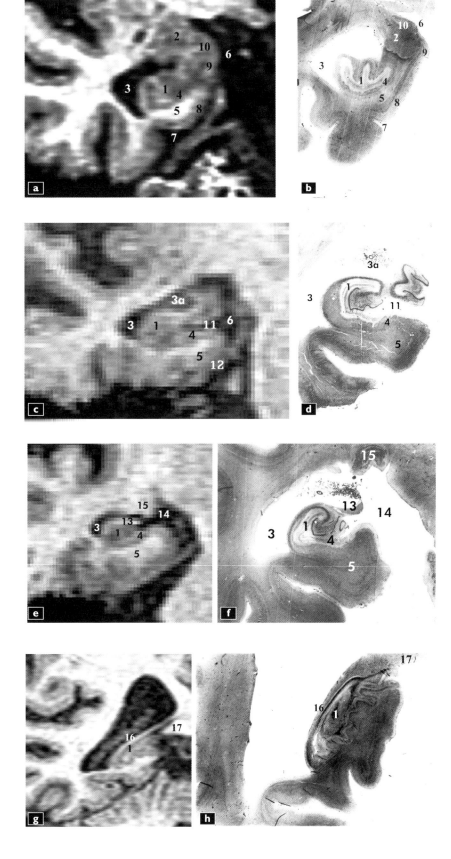

Figure 1 (a–h) Postmortem histology sections stained with cresyl violet and T1 weighted *in vivo* MRI coronal images depicting the normal anatomy of the hippocampal region

Ammonis (hippocampus proper) has three major layers: the stratum oriens, the stratum pyramidale, and a multi-strata layer comprising the radiatum, lacunosum and moleculare strata. Aspects of these layers can be appreciated using MRI (Figure 2). On the basis of the types of the pyramidal neurons, the cornu Ammonis can be divided into four sectors: CA1 to CA4.

CSF anatomy of the hippocampus

Cerebrospinal fluid covers a large part of the hippocampal surface area and marks some of its boundaries. This includes the temporal horn of the lateral ventricle and a complex of CSF-containing fissures and cisterns. Figures 3a, b and c depict, in three orthogonal planes, the orientation of the transverse fissure relative to the hippocampus, parahippocampal gyrus, thalamic structures and ventricular CSF. These CSF landmarks are of particular interest for *in vivo* imaging as they provide high-contrast boundaries between the hippocampus and surrounding structures such as the thalamus. In addition, increases in these CSF spaces reflect regional tissue atrophy and they are therefore of interest in the clinical evaluation. In the coronal view (Figure 3, top panel), the lateral boundaries of the transverse fissure of Bichat (also known as the lateral transverse fissure (LTF)) is the medial aspect of the dentate gyrus (DG) and the fimbria (Fi). The coronal view best permits separation of the choroidal (CF) and hippocampal fissure (HF) extensions of the LTF. In the horizontal or axial view, the LTF begins at the posterior border of the pes hippocampus or uncus (Un) (see Figure 3, middle panel). Medially the LTF communicates with the

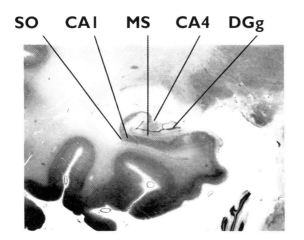

Postmortem

a

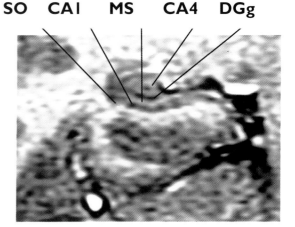

MRI

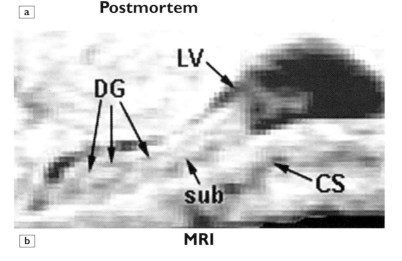

b   **MRI**

Figure 2 Postmortem histological slice (a) and corresponding high-resolution coronal MRI image (b) through the hippocampal body, depicting: the alveus and the stratum oriens (SO); stratum pyramidale of the CA1 (CA1); a multi-strata layer comprising the stratum radiatum, lacunosum and moleculare of the cornu Ammonis, and the molecular layer of the dentate gyrus (MS); the granule layer of the dentate gyrus (DGg); and the sector CA4 (CA4). (c) Imaging of the long axis of the dentate gyrus in a sagittal plane

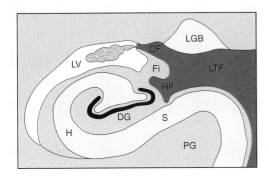

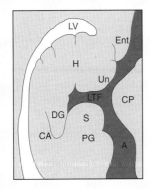

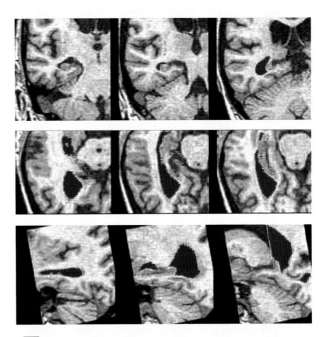

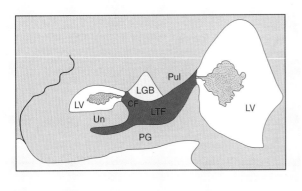

a

b

Figure 3 (a) Schematic representations of coronal (top left panel), axial (middle left panel) and sagittal (bottom left panel) views of the hippocampal region. CF, choroid fissure recess; CP, cerebral peduncle; H, hippocampus; HF, hippocampal fissure; LGB, lateral geniculate body; LTF, lateral transverse fissure; LV, lateral ventricle, PG, parahippocampal gyrus; Pul, pulvinar; S, subiculum; TC, tela choroidea. (b) The MRI scans were obtained on a General Electric Advantage 1.5T imager using a spoiled gradient echo sequece of 35/9/1 (TR/TE/Excitations), a 60° flip angle, an 18-cm field of view and a 256×128 acquisition matrix. We obtained 124 contiguous coronal images with a slice thickness of 1.3 mm. On 56 of these images, using a two-fold image magnification to aid in region drawing (pixel size=0.35 mm), we outlined and coded in red the hippocampal fissures, including the transverse fissure of Bichat, the choroidal fissure and the hippocampal fissure. Also the CSF of the lateral ventricle was outlined and coded in blue. Figure 3b (top right panel) shows three of the 56 slices coded. All 56 coronal images and the coded regions were reformatted and displayed as 5-mm contiguous slices in a negative angulation axial plan (Figure 3b middle right panel) and in a sagittal plane (Figure 3b bottom right panel). The reformatted axial images and sagittal images depict the anatomical relationship of the two CSF compartments

ambient cistern (A), which borders the cerebral peduncles (CP). Both the coronal and sagittal planes (Figure 3, bottom panel) of section permit identification of the structures bounding the ventral surface of the transverse fissure, namely the subiculum (S) of the parahippocampal gyrus (PG), as well as the identification of those thalamic structures bounding the dorsal margin, the lateral geniculate body (LGB) and the pulvinar (Pul).

Subicular complex

The subicular complex is divided into three parts: the subiculum proper, presubiculum and parasubiculum. Subicular complex subdivisions comprise two layers: the molecular and the pyramidal layers. In the presubiculum, a third layer, the parvopyramidal layer, is distinguished between the molecular and the pyramidal layers. At present, there is no reported strategy to distinguish between these layers using MRI techniques.

Entorhinal cortex

The entorhinal cortex and the transentorhinal cortex form a major part of the anterior parahippocampal gyrus. Phylogenetically, they are relatively old structures. Based on histology and connectivity, the entorhinal cortex is transitional between the hippocampus and the neocortex. The term entorhinal cortex was introduced by Brodmann[12] as a synonym for his area 28. Subsequent studies divided the entorhinal cortex into many fields[13,14] and increased the number to as many as 23 different fields[15]. Recent cytoarchitectonic studies showed that parcellation of the entorhinal cortex in humans is largely parallel to that in the monkey and distinguish only eight different fields[16,17]. However, to date little is known about the physiological function and the consequences of pathology in these fields.

The entorhinal cortex is made up of six layers[8,17]. Layer II is one of the most outstanding and distinguishing areas of the entorhinal cortex and is made up of islands of large modified pyramidal and stellate cells. Some of these islands are large enough to be appreciated grossly. As compared with the neocortex, one of the most characteristic features of the entorhinal cortex in all species is the absence of an internal granular layer. In its place is an acellular layer of dense fibers called the lamina dissecans.

The entorhinal cortex is adjacent to the more lateral perirhinal cortex (areas 35 and 36 of Brodmann). There is no clear-cut border between area 35 and the entorhinal cortex. These two fields appear to have an obliquely oriented boundary, where the deep layers of the entorhinal cortex extend somewhat more laterally than the superficial layers. This distinctly angled border between area 35 and the entorhinal cortex has been emphasized by Braak[18], who has labelled the region of overlap the transentorhinal cortex. With serial coronal MRI sections, one can reliably identify gyral landmarks that serve as the approximate boundaries for the entorhinal cortex region. These landmarks include, on the medial surface, the semilunar gyrus and the sulcus semianularis. The lateral boundary is approximated at anterior levels by the rhinal sulcus and posteriorly by the collateral sulcus (see Figures 1a and b).

Hippocampal formation connections

The entorhinal cortex, the gateway to the hippocampus, receives massive synaptic input from neocortical association areas and less pronounced input from primary sensory areas[19,20]. In addition, it receives input from many subcortical regions, including the midbrain raphe nuclei, the ventral tegmental area, the locus coeruleus, the septum, the thalamus and hypothalamus, the amygdala, the magnocellular basal forebrain nuclei and the claustrum[21]. The entorhinal cortex provides the major source of afferent information to the hippocampus via the perforant path[22]. The predominant component of the perforant path has been regarded as the projection from the stellate layer II neurons of the entorhinal cortex which synapse in the molecular layer on the dendrites of the granular cells of the dentate gyrus. In the classical model of the trisynaptic circuit, this is the first link, followed by the mossy fiber connections to CA3 pyramidal cells and completed by the Schaffer collateral input to CA1. This simplified circuit diagram has been modified recently as it has been shown that there is actually a second distinct projection from the entorhinal cortex, the alternative perforant pathway, that contributes fibers to all the hippocampal fields and to the subiculum[22]. The alternative perforant pathway is formed by projection from neurons of layers II and III of the entorhinal cortex to the subiculum, CA1, CA2 and CA3. Much hippocampal output is also directed back to the entorhinal cortex and neocortex directly from the CA1 and via relays in the subiculum. Thus, the entorhinal cortex occupies the key position with respect to gating the interactions, output as well as input, between the hippocampus and the rest of the brain.

Neuropathology

Hippocampal atrophy in AD

Impairment of memory is one of the earliest features of AD. Clinical symptoms slowly increase in severity and are accompanied by personality changes, deterioration of language functions and involvement of the extrapyramidal motor system[23]. Disease severity is associated with a hierarchy of pathological changes progressing from the entorhinal cortex and hippocampus to involvement of the neocortex[5]. Postmortem histopathological studies show that the hippocampal formation, especially the entorhinal and transentorhinal cortex, is one of the earliest and most affected structures in AD[5,24]. Morphological studies of the hippocampal formation reveal neurofibrillary changes and granulovacuolar degeneration of neurons, synaptic and neuronal loss and β-amyloid deposition in plaques and vascular walls[5,25]. Neurofibrillary degeneration and the loss of projection neurons responsible for the majority of afferent and efferent connections of the hippocampal formation cause both the disruption of intrahippocampal connections and functional isolation of the hippocampal formation from other parts of the memory system[24]. Neuronal loss in the hippocampal formation appears to be a major component of the memory impairment seen in AD[24,26]. Neurofibrillary degeneration has been put forth as a cause of neuronal loss and atrophy of the hippocampal formation[24,26–28]. The later onset of amyloid deposits in the hippocampal formation subdivisions and the topographical differences in distribution and number have suggested that amyloid and neurofibrillary changes develop independently[29]. The impact of amyloid deposits on hippocampal formation atrophy is not known.

The severe atrophy of the hippocampal formation in AD is found, to a similar extent, in both cellular and fiber layers[27,30]. In a recent study of five controls and 13 severe AD patients, the AD patients showed marked volume losses in the pyramidal layer of the cornu Ammonis (61%), in the stratum radiatum (74%) and in the lacunosum/moleculare (66%)[30]. The volumetric loss of the pyramidal layer reflects the loss of pyramidal cells, whereas the decrease in volume of the stratum radiatum and lacunosum/moleculare encompasses the loss of, first, apical dendrites of the pyramidal cells and, second, the perforant fibers and Schaffer collaterals. In the subicular complex, severe AD patients also showed a 68% volumetric loss of the pyramidal layer. This volume loss is a direct effect of loss of cell bodies and perineuronal processes. The atrophy of the apical dendrites of pyramidal cells and of the dense network of fibers running through the molecular layer of the subicular complex probably accounts for the 54% decrement in the volume of this layer. The dentate gyrus was the only hippocampal subdivision that did not manifest significant volumetric decrement relative to control subjects. The granular layer is known to be mostly spared in the course of AD and is affected by neurofibrillary pathology only in late-stage AD[5]. In this study, neuronal counts were not made in the entorhinal cortex.

In another pathologic study[30], the volume of the hippocampal formation subdivisions was examined for its relationship to both the stage (as determined by the functional assessment staging procedure (FAST) scale[31]) and the duration of AD. Using the FAST scale, the following relationships were observed with regional volume measures: CA1 ($r=-0.79$, $p<0.01$) subiculum ($r=-0.75$, $p<0.001$), and entorhinal cortex ($r=-0.62$, $p<0.05$). Figure 4 schematically depicts the average histologically derived hippocampal (cornu Ammonis) and subicular volumes for the normal elderly and the AD patient groups.

Over the estimated duration of clinically manifest AD, we estimated an overall decrease of 60% in the volume of the hippocampal formation. These volumetric decreases in the cornu Ammonis, subicular

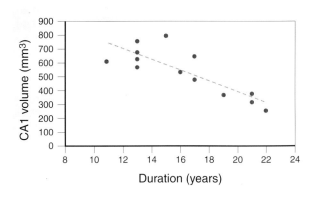

Figure 5 Scattergram plotting volume of the CA1 against disease duration

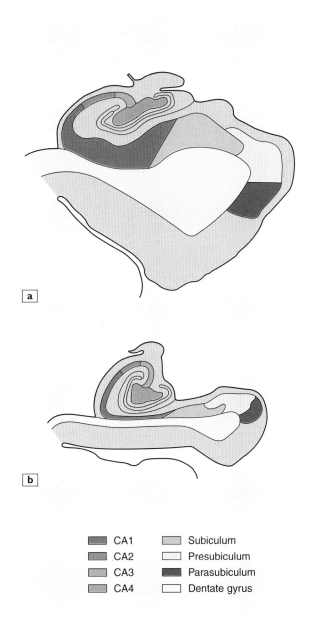

■ CA1	▨ Subiculum
▨ CA2	▢ Presubiculum
▨ CA3	■ Parasubiculum
▨ CA4	▢ Dentate gyrus

Figure 4 Schematic drawings of histologically derived volumes of the hippocampus and subicular complex. (a) From the average normal control; (b) from the average AD patient

complex and the entorhinal cortex were 64, 70, and 51%, respectively. These cross-sectionally derived results suggest that changes occur in the hippocampal formation and most of its structural components throughout the course of AD (Figure 5). Direct evi-

dence for the patterns and rate of progressive regional atrophy requires *in vivo* neuroimaging.

Determination of the subvolumes of the whole hippocampal formation and estimation of the total number of neurons, neurofibrillary tangles and amyloid deposits in these volumes enabled relationships to be analyzed between lesion counts, neuronal number and the volume of the hippocampal subdivisions[27]. Specifically, the volume in the hippocampus proper, as determined by either histological criteria or postmortem MRI studies, correlated linearly with number of neurons ($r=0.83$, $p<0.01$, Figure 6a). This finding, as well as the observation that the volume of the hippocampus as determined by MRI reflects the actual size of the structure (M. Bobinski and colleagues, unpublished data) (Figure 6b), is of particular relevance to *in vivo* neuroimaging. These data add support to the contention that *in vivo* neuroimaging measurements of atrophy reflect actual histological damage and neuron loss.

Moreover, among all the neurons counted, we observed that the percentage of remaining neurons with neurofibrillary changes was correlated with the estimated neuronal loss ($r=0.73$, $p<0.05$). This suggests that neurofibrillary pathology is a possible etiological factor in neuronal and volumetric loss in the hippocampal formation of AD patients. On the other hand, no significant relationships were found between either neuronal counts or volumes of the hippocampal formation subdivisions and the numerical density of plaques, or the total number of

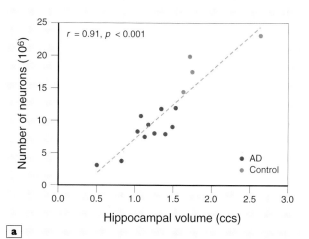

a

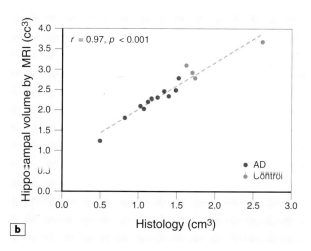

b

Figure 6 Scattergrams depicting the relationships between (a) the hippocampal volume and the hippocampal neuronal counts; and (b) the MRI-determined volume of the hippocampus and the volume as determined from the histology sections

plaques, or the area occupied by amyloid or the density of vessels with amyloid angiopathy. Therefore, the data indicate that, unlike tangle pathology, plaque pathology may not be associated with neuronal loss.

AD-related neuronal loss

Neuronal loss in the hippocampal formation in AD has been described by many authors. The entorhinal cortex, CA1 and subiculum are consistently severely affected, while the granular layer of the dentate gyrus is generally spared[28,32,33]. Studies of the hip-

pocampus proper show that the number of subdivisions that are found to evidence neuronal loss depends to a great extent on the duration of the illness and/or the clinical stage of AD in the patients investigated[26]. For those individuals clinically least affected, significant neuronal loss was observed in the CA1 and subiculum. For the group of patients with more severe AD, significant neuronal loss was observed in the CA1, CA2, CA3, CA4 and the subiculum. Recent studies of the entorhinal cortex add to our understanding by demonstrating clear evidence for early neuronal loss[32].

Despite the complex connectivity in the hippocampal formation, neurofibrillary pathology and neuronal loss appear to develop in a structure-specific fashion. Braak and Braak described a staging scheme (see Chapter 5) of neurofibrillary changes in the brain based on the temporal and topographical distribution of these lesions[5]. According to these authors, neurofibrillary changes develop first in the transentorhinal cortex, then in the entorhinal cortex (transentorhinal stages). Further progression involves the CA1, the subiculum and the CA4, then sectors CA2 and CA3 of the cornu Ammonis and the parvopyramidal layer of the presubiculum. This was referred to as the limbic stage of pathology. The changes in the dentate gyrus and all isocortical association areas (neocortex) appear in the last stage of this classification, the so-called isocortical stages.

West and co-workers who, using unbiased stereological techniques, estimated the total numbers of neurons in several hippocampal formation subdivisions[33], also reported structure-specific neuronal loss in AD. Among normals they found neuronal losses in two subdivisions, the hilus (CA4) and the subiculum. In the AD group, they also observed additional loss of neurons in the CA1. Therefore, the pathology of AD does not simply reflect an acceleration of normal aging. The regional pattern of neuronal loss in AD is qualitatively and quantitatively different from that observed in normal aging.

We carried out a stereology study on the brains of 11 AD patients with moderate, moderately severe, or severe dementia, and five normal controls. In this study, we examined both the numbers of neurons and neurofibrillary tangles in the hippocampus[26].

We found that the CA1 sector was severely affected by neurofibrillary pathology and neuronal loss. In this sector, we found that there was a profound loss of neurons (86%) and that 71% of the surviving neurons were affected by neurofibrillary changes. The subiculum showed somewhat less pathology: the neuronal loss was 68%, and 52% of surviving neurons were affected by neurofibrillary pathology. Other structures, such as CA2, CA3 and CA4, are much less affected. They showed neuronal losses of 75%, 53% and 55%, respectively and neurofibrillary pathology in 33%, 26% and 28% of surviving neurons, respectively. Finally, the granular layer of the dentate gyrus was the only hippocampal subdivision without significant neuronal loss over the course of AD. This surprising finding either may reflect a unique lack of vulnerability of these cells or perhaps is related to increased cellular plasticity in this region. In the AD group, only 4% of neurons in the granular layer of the dentate gyrus showed neurofibrillary changes. Overall, these results support the hypothesis that there is a selective pattern of neuronal vulnerability in AD.

Postmortem studies have documented the presence of NFTs in the entorhinal cortex and transentorhinal cortex of non-demented elderly individuals[34]. In the brains of early-stage AD subjects, neurofibrillary changes are always detectable in the entorhinal cortex and transentorhinal cortex. Consequently, pathology limited to the entorhinal cortex and transentorhinal cortex may represent a clinically silent phase of the disease[34]. Neurons of layer II and IV are particularly susceptible to degeneration. Eventually during the course of AD, virtually all neurons in layer II contain NFTs[5,24,35–37]. Layer II is also the first cortical layer showing the presence of ghost tangles (clusters of extracellular filaments which are remnants of a degenerated neuron)[5]. Layer IV is affected after layer II. Only a comparatively few NFTs are found in layers III and V, and these usually develop late in the course of AD[5].

It has been suggested that the degeneration of much of the neuronal architecture of the entorhinal cortex destroys a large functional part of hippocampal input and output and that this destruction results in the memory and cognitive deficits associated with the early stages of AD[24]. In a detailed stereological study, Gomez-Isla and associates[32] found that subjects with very mild cognitive impairment (clinical dementia rating (CDR)=0.5) had 32% fewer neurons in the entorhinal cortex than controls. In layer II, neuronal loss reached 60%. In severe dementia cases (CDR=3), the total number of neurons in layer II decreased by 90% and in layer IV by 70%. Moreover, neuronal numbers were negatively correlated with tangle and plaque densities. Their study showed that a significant neuronal loss in layer II of the entorhinal cortex distinguished even very mild AD from non-demented aging[32].

In summary, modern stereological techniques have recently shown that the CA1 of the hippocampus and layers II and IV of the entorhinal cortex are the most vulnerable to AD pathology and are potentially specific for AD[32,33]. Combined with traditional semiquantitative neuropathological techniques for estimating the number and distribution of lesions, the data suggest a pattern of alterations that define the hippocampal formation as anatomy that is vulnerable in the early stages of AD.

Hippocampal formation pathology in normal aging

Studies of normal elderly people typically show that NFT accumulation in the entorhinal cortex and/or hippocampus dramatically increases with increasing age[6,38–40]. It is informative that strong age relationships remain despite methodological differences in patient recruitment, cognitive evaluation, staining procedures and anatomical sampling. These differences across studies appear more likely to affect the absolute numbers of affected individuals rather than the brain regions or the relative numbers of patients affected across the studied age groups. For example, Giannakopoulos and co-workers[6] examined 1131 brains of normal and mildly affected but non-demented elderly people derived from a hospital-based medical and surgical service. They observed NFTs in the CA1 of the hippocampus in 25% of the sample. By comparison, NFTs were uncommon in these patients in the superior frontal (4%) and occipital cortices (3%). Langui and colleagues[39] examined the entorhinal cortex and hippocampus from 167 brains of normal subjects. The diagnosis of normal was based on clinical notes; no cognitive testing was performed. They observed that AD changes (NFT or senile plaques) were found in less than 20% of subjects under 60 years of age, in over 80% of individuals between 60 and 80 years and in nearly 100% of the 56 subjects over 80 years of age. The predominant form of pathology was the NFT, either alone or frequently in combination with senile plaques. Only 2% of normal brains showed senile plaques in the absence of NFTs. Summarizing over several other studies that examined the hippocampal formation along with neocortical sites, there appears to be a strong trend for non-demented subjects to show an age-related tendency towards NFT accumulation that is concentrated in the hippocampal formation[38,40,41]. Although senile plaques also tend to accumulate with age, typically plaques accumulate at greater ages and have a preference for the neocortex rather than the hippocampal formation[6,38]. These data, which support the Braak model, suggest that age-associated hippocampal formation lesions represent the earliest lesions associated with AD. Moreover, it appears that in association with these early lesions there is a reduction in the volume of the affected tissue, thus making this observation a target for early diagnosis using *in vivo* neuroimging. It was reported that normal elderly individuals with NFT lesions in the hippocampus showed hippocampal volume reductions when compared with normal age-matched elderly individuals without NFT[42]. It therefore appears that the inverse relationship between NFT deposition and hippocampal volume extends throughout the range of normal to severely demented AD. Such neuropathology findings encourage the more comprehensive *in vivo* examination of the hippocampal formation in aging and AD.

Neuropsychology

Perirhinal and entorhinal ablation studies

Because of their unique location and connections with the hippocampus, the perirhinal cortex (also referred to in the human as transentorhinal cortex[43]) and the entorhinal cortex[44] have long been considered as candidate structures in mediating memory[45,46]. The current view describes the perirhinal

and entorhinal regions as providing the major input to the hippocampus *via* the perforant pathway. There is virtually a complete absence of literature on the human neuropsychology of entorhinal cortex lesions. However, given that there is a reasonably close homology between the human and the non-human primate entorhinal cortexes[8,47], we will briefly concentrate on the literature on the lesions of the non-human primate. Ablation studies damaging variable amounts of entorhinal cortex and perirhinal cortex demonstrated disruption of recognition memory for complex shapes presented tactually[48–50] and impairments in complex visual tasks such as facial discrimination[45,51]. These lesions do not appear to affect perceptual functioning. In one study, combining damage to the entorhinal and perirhinal regions with damage to the amygdala produced deficits in visual recognition that were equivalent to removal of the entire hippocampal formation and the amygdala[52]. This result suggested that the lesions deafferented the hippocampus. Suzuki and associates[53] showed that perirhinal lesions and parahippocampal gyrus lesions (largely sparing the entorhinal cortex and hippocampus) produced severe and permanent memory (non-matching to sample) deficits on both visual and tactual object memory tests that were increased with increasing delays[54]. These data suggested that the perirhinal cortex may directly contribute to memory processing. Relatedly, other studies have suggested that perirhinal lesions can be more damaging to memory performance than hippocampal lesions[52] or entorhinal lesions[55,56].

In a recent review of the literature on both primates and rats, Suzuki[57] concluded that the perirhinal cortex participates in a broad range of memory-related functions including recognition memory, associative memory, emotional memory and consolidation functions. A less clear view has emerged for the entorhinal cortex. Ablation of the entorhinal cortex in one study produced temporary deficits. The reversibility of deficits suggests either that the structure is not essential for learning and memory[58], or that the structure may be protected by a redundancy of connections, possibly by an alternative perforant pathway[59,60]. Further evidence complicating our understanding comes from recent studies examining the effects of entorhinal cortex lesions on the hippocampus. Experimental studies in the primate report that entorhinal lesions cause a loss of hippocampal CA3 neurons[61], an observation also reported in the human following infarction of the entorhinal cortex[62]; in the rat they cause reductions in measures of hippocampal cholinergic integrity[63]. In contrast to the uncertainty regarding the key sites within the hippocampal formation mediating memory encoding and consolidation, primate ablation experiments clearly show that the severity of memory deficits increase as the amount of damaged tissue increases from a perirhinal locus to include the entorhinal cortex, hippocampus and subiculum[53,54,56]. These observations are provocative in the light of the estimated pattern of progressive hippocampal formation lesions and memory changes in early AD, and point to the opportunity of observing these evolving brain–behavior relationships *in vivo* and in the human.

Memory performance in normal aging and AD

Cross-sectional human studies have reported that the functions most vulnerable to aging are those involving memory[64], sensory motor processing and attention[65,66], visuospatial function, praxis[67], and abstraction/problem solving[65,67]. In an important contribution, Ivnik and colleagues[68] studied 394 normal subjects over the age of 55 years. Their normative data showed an age-related decline in learning and memory on verbally presented items from the Auditory–Verbal Learning Test. Consistent age effects were seen for items recalled after interference and after a 30-min delay. Evidence from longitudinal normal aging studies of relatively short duration (1–4 years) suggests that performance declines in the elderly in verbal working memory (requiring the short term storage and manipulation of information prior to responding), speed-dependent tasks, world knowledge, vigilance, learning and problem solving[69–74]. The anatomical basis for these performance changes remains essentially unknown as these studies have typically not included neuroimaging.

For many years it has been recognized that memory impairments are the most reliable clinical symptom in early AD. However, relatively few normal elderly people demonstrate decline in delayed recall performance measures in short-interval longitudinal normal aging studies[75]. This observation led to the development of several tests predicting future AD with reasonably high diagnostic specificity. These successful measures included delayed verbal recall tasks[76–83], and object recognition memory with delayed recall[84–87]. Other promising diagnostic tests include measures of verbal fluency and semantic knowledge[77,87,88]. For example, Fuld and associates[85] demonstrated that, among 474 normal elderly patients, the delayed recall and recognition of ten objects separately presented tactually followed by visual naming predicted dementia over ≤ 2 years in 56 patients (12%) with a sensitivity of 59% and a specificity of 94%. Bondi and colleagues[76] reported that elderly normal subjects with family histories of dementia performed more poorly at baseline on verbal delayed recall tasks than elderly subjects without family histories. Over a 2-year interval, four out of 24 (17%) subjects with a positive family history declined to either MCI or AD as compared with none out of 25 individuals with a negative family history. The baseline verbal delayed recall measures distinguished between declining and non-declining individuals. Performance on the modified Wisconsin Card Sorting Test and the Grooved Pegboard Test did not discriminate the decliners. In our laboratory, we observed that list learning and object function tests showed the best sensitivity and specificity (85–90%) for the prediction of decline[84].

Overall, the anatomical basis for the reduced baseline delayed recall performance that forms the basis of the predictive tests remains poorly understood. Extrapolating to the human condition from non-human primate studies, the evidence suggests that medial temporal lobe lesions cause impairments in declarative memory performance under conditions of delayed recall[46]. Some of these same relationships are beginning to emerge in the human aging literature with neuroimaging of the hippocampal formation.

In summary, the neuropathology and the neuropsychology data independently offer excellent justification for examining the integrity of the hippocampal formation as a potentially informative anatomy to evaluate the transition between normal aging and AD-related memory decline. However, efficient memory functioning is based not only on the integrity of the hippocampal formation. Many different locations of brain damage have been associated with memory dysfunctions[89], and generalized atrophic changes that are known to occur in normal aged individuals may also contribute to memory changes[90]. Consequently, the determination of meaningful brain–memory relationships in aging humans requires both qualitative and quantitative characterization of the cognitive deficits as well as examination of the anatomic specificity of any statistically significant brain–memory relationship.

Neuroimaging studies of the hippocampal formation

In the late 1980s, several laboratories nearly simultaneously reported that the hippocampal region could be reliably studied with structural neuroimaging[91-95]. This advance was partly facilitated by the availability of MRI. Thus, numerous research efforts were directed away from more general markers of brain atrophy (ventricular size and cortical atrophy) to anatomically better defined regional assessments. In the AD literature a growing consensus exists among *in vivo* neuroimaging studies regarding the involvement of the hippocampus. All studies report increased hippocampal atrophy relative to age-matched controls. These results are reflected in measures of parenchymal volume[7,93,95-102]; qualitative ratings of the amount of CSF accumulating in the hippocampal fissures[91,92,103,104], linear two-dimensional estimates of hippocampal width[105,106], measures of medial temporal lobe gray matter volume[107], the size of the suprasellar cistern[108], and the distance between the right and left uncus (see reference 109 for review). However, before hippocampal atrophy can be considered a diagnostic marker for early (preclinical) AD, several lines of investigation need to be further developed. Specifically, we need to improve our understanding of the prevalence and severity of hippocampal atrophy over the stages of AD, and as a function of age, gender and genetic factors. The diagnostic specificity of hippocampal atrophy for AD needs to be established, and the relationship between the atrophy deter-mined by imaging and neuropathological features of the disease needs to be validated. Moreover, very little is known of the longitudinal course of AD from the standpoint of structural neuroimaging. Only a small number of studies have investigated changes over two or three time points. Nevertheless, a considerable body of information has accumulated that strongly suggests the continuation and further development of these efforts.

Below we review our clinical structural neuroimaging studies of the hippocampal formation. These cross-sectional and longitudinal studies show that imaging of the hippocampal formation is of potential use in the early detection and diagnosis of age-related memory changes, and in the prediction of future dementia and a diagnosis of AD. Moreover, these preliminary *in vivo* data support the Braak model, which proposes the staging of the brain involvement of AD. In this model, the earliest stages of AD are marked by selective involvement of the entorhinal cortex followed by a hippocampal stage and finally by progressive neocortical pathology.

Studies of the hippocampus

Cross-sectional hippocampal studies of normal aging and AD

Over a decade ago, prior to the availability of MRI, the first imaging studies of the hippocampal region were conducted using X-ray computed tomography (CT). Limited by the range of gantry rotation, axial plane rather than coronal plane images were acquired. As opposed to MRI, where there is sufficient soft tissue contrast to identify gray matter structures, with CT the optimal contrast is between brain and CSF. In order to maximize the amount of the hippocampus visible on any single axial slice, we developed a CT plane of acquisition to parallel the long axis of the hippocampus, resulting in a so-called negative angulation view[92]. With the negative angulation view, one can observe the transverse and the associated choroidal–hippocampal fissures as a continuous CSF space that enlarges with volume loss in the hippocampus and subiculum. Our protocol utilized a 4-mm-thick slice, which provided us with 1–3 slices going though the CSF accumulations that would show atrophic hippocampal changes. Moreover, as these procedures and the qualitative decisions were easy to carry out, it was possible to examine large numbers of subjects.

In our first CT studies of the hippocampal region, we used a qualitative four-point assessment scale to rate the extent of the CSF accumulation as seen with the negative angulation. This qualitative measure was validated against the actual hippocampal volume[96], and so is referred to as a measure of hippocampal atrophy. The hippocampal atrophy scale points included: 0=no atrophy, 1=questionable, 2=mild and 3=moderate to severe. The cut-off rating of definite atrophy, which corresponded to a rating of ≥2 in either hemisphere, was used to define definite hippocampal atrohpy (see Figure 7).

For our first study, we developed a negative angle protocol to examine the hippocampal region in aging and AD. In this study and the studies below, all study participants underwent an extensive research protocol of medical, neurological, psychiatric and neuropsychologic examinations. These examinations were used to exclude from the study individuals with evidence of conditions other than AD that could affect brain functioning or structure, and to include individuals with changes presumably only related to age or AD. We examined 175

subjects[91]. The results of this study demonstrated that hippocampal atrophy was typically found in AD independent of age and disease severity. Moreover, in a longitudinal sample of MCI patients, hippocampal atrophy was predictive of future dementia.

More recently, we studied 405 patients[103]. Four clinical groups were defined using NINCDS/ADRDA criteria and the Global Deterioration Scores (GDS)[23]. The groups identified included normal elderly (GDS 1 and 2; $n=130$), mild AD (GDS 4; $n=73$) and moderate to severe AD (GDS 5 and 6; $n=130$). The fourth group, the minimal impairment group (MCI; n=72), was defined as having GDS=3 and Mini-Mental State Exam (MMSE) scores >23[110].

A second validation component of this study showed that hippocampal atrophy was equivalently determined with CT and MRI (T_1 weighted 4-mm-thick axial images). The clinical data showed that hippocampal atrophy was significantly more prevalent in all clinical groups as compared with controls. Hippocampal atrophy was shown in 78% of the MCI (GDS=3), 84% of the mild AD (GDS=4) and 96% of the moderate to severe AD (GDS≥5) groups. Controls showed hippocampal atrophy in 29% of subjects (Figure 8).

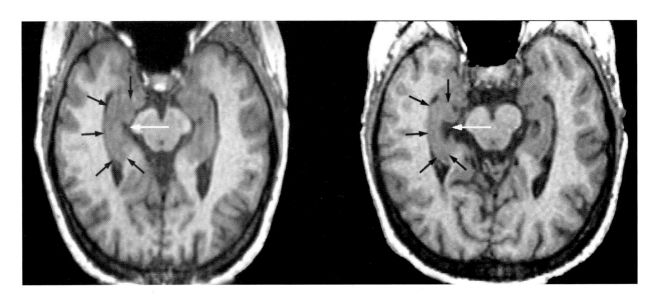

Figure 7 Axial MRI scans depicting the hippocampal area from a normal control (left) and an age-matched AD patient (right). Scans highlight the qualitative assessment for hippocampal atrophy

The same study showed that normal controls showed a striking age dependence of hippocampal atrophy while the cognitively impaired groups showed prevalence rates independent of age (Figure 9).

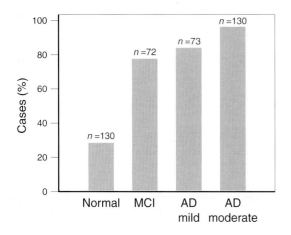

Figure 8 The prevalence of hippocampal atrophy in four groups (n=405): normal elderly, minimally impaired elderly (MCI) and two AD with different severity levels of cognitive impairment (mild and moderate)

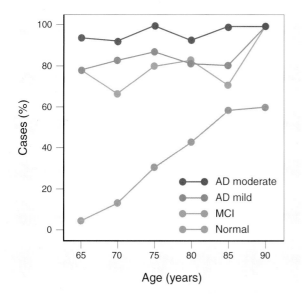

Figure 9 The prevalence of hippocampal atrophy for normal, minimal and two levels of AD as a function of age (n=405)

Longitudinal studies predicting the development of dementia

The results of our cross-sectional studies of hippocampal atrophy showed that hippocampal changes occur with a high frequency in MCI patients known to be at high risk for AD[84]. We therefore reasoned that hippocampal atrophy might be predictive of deterioration to symptoms consistent with the course of AD. In order to assess the prognostic value of hippocampal changes, a 4-year follow-up CT study was carried out in a normal elderly group (n=54, aged 70±8 years) and an MCI group (n=32, aged 71±9 years)[104]. Over the interval, 23 (72%) of the MCI group and two (4%) of the normal elderly group deteriorated to receive the diagnosis of AD (GDS≥4). For the MCI group, baseline hippocampal atrophy was present in 91% of the declining group and in 11% of the non-declining group. The results also showed that the prediction of decline was not related to age, as equal numbers of the decliners came from the groups above and below 75 years of age. No differences were found between the percentages of males and females that declined. Both cortical sulcal prominence and ventricular enlargement at baseline were related to the observation of decline. However, as compared with the overall prediction accuracies of 91% for hippocampal atrophy, cortical sulcal prominence and ventricular enlargement measures yielded overall prediction accuracy scores of 70% and 69%, respectively. In summary, the relatively high accuracy of hippocampal atrophy for the prediction of decline, and the high rate of preservation in the group not showing hippocampal atrophy, suggest the unique potential of hippocampal atrophy in the clinical examination of early AD.

The results of these studies pointed to the need for longitudinal study of the temporal relationship between hippocampal atrophy, neocortical atrophy and the development of intellectual dysfunction. As only 4% of our normal elderly sample deteriorated to dementia while 15% had baseline hippocampal atrophy, this study also suggested that, in order to evaluate the predictive risk of hippocampal atrophy carefully, the following are necessary: first, we must extend beyond the 4 years the period of observation;

second, we must use more sensitive indices of hippocampal integrity; and third, we must utilize assessments of neuropsychological performance that are more fine grained.

The anatomic specificity of hippocampal volume loss in patients at risk for AD

A central requirement in the development of a biological marker is to establish the relationship between the marker and the pathological substrate that characterizes the disease. Some recent evidence suggests that hippocampal atrophy may actually meet some of the requirements as a marker for AD. One study reported that normal elderly individuals with NFT lesions in the hippocampus showed hippocampal volume reductions when compared with normal age-matched elderly individuals without NFT[42]. In an MRI–neuropathology validation study, we first examined, using postmortem brain tissue (fixed for a minimum of 3 weeks in formalin), the relationship between the histologically derived hippocampal volume and the MRI-derived hippocampal volume. Second, we examined the relationship between the estimated volumes and the numbers of hippocampal neurons using unbiased counting techniques. The results from the volume study showed that the methods produced virtually equivalent results ($n=16$, $r=0.97$, $p<0.001$; Figure 6b)[111]. The results from the neuron counting study showed that the total number of counted neurons was strongly related to both the MRI-based hippocampal volume and the histology-based volume ($r=0.90$, $p<0.001$; Figure 6). Overall, these findings indicate significant relationships between the magnitude of AD-related neuropathology and the hippocampal volume. Particularly intriguing is the fact that the relationships appear to extend throughout the range of clinical severity for AD that includes cognitively normal elderly individuals at one extreme and those with confirmed clinical AD at the other.

Using MRI volume data, we investigated the hypothesis that hippocampal volume reductions are the most consistently observed gross structural phenomena in the early stages of AD. We predicted that the hippocampal volume would be superior to neo-

cortical tissue volumes in the diagnositic classification of MCI patients. We also predicted that the neocortical volumes would be significantly reduced in cases with clinically determined AD. To address these issues, a volumetric MRI and neuropsychological study of 27 normal elderly people, 22 elderly MCI patients and 27 AD patients was conducted[97]. We used 4-mm-thick T_1-weighted coronal MRI images. Here, we measured five major anatomically defined regions encompassing the entire temporal lobe, starting anteriorly from the level of the posterior pes hippocampus and ending posteriorly at the level of the splenium of the corpus callosum. The regions included the hippocampus, the parahippocampal gyrus, the fusiform gyrus, the superior temporal gyrus and the combined middle and inferior temporal gyri. All groups were matched for age, gender and education. As compared with the normal elderly group, the MCI patients showed a 14% volume loss that was anatomically specific to the hippocampus (Table 1). The AD group, on the other hand, showed significant differences relative to the normal group for all temporal lobe volumes. The reduction in the hippocampus was 22% and, in the neocortical regions, the reductions ranged from 9 to 20%. In the MCI group, these data also demonstrated an anatomically unique relationship between hippocampus volume and delayed recall performance. In addition, because the entire temporal lobe was studied, these data additionally supported the hypothesis that the hippocampal–delayed recall relationship is anatomically specific.

Table I Regional MRI data on parenchymal volume changes (%) relative to controls for the group with mild cognitive impairments (MCI) and the group with Alzheimer's disease (AD)

	MCI	AD
Hippocampus	−14	−22
Parahippocampal gyrus	—	−14
Fusiform gyrus	—	−20
Middle/inferior temporal gyri	—	−9
Superior temporal gyrus	—	−10

When the MCI group was contrasted with the AD group, this study also clearly showed that lateral temporal lobe volume losses were necessary to classify cases with dementia correctly. With the use of logistic regression to classify the MCI and AD patients, the lateral temporal lobe measurements were found significantly to add, over and above the hippocampus and the parahippocampal gyrus (medial temporal lobe), to the classification accuracy. The medial temporal lobe volume correctly classified 67% of patients and inclusion of the lateral regions raised this value to 80%. In the classification of normal and AD patients, the medial temporal lobe correctly classified 87% and with addition of the lateral temporal lobe the correct classification significantly improved to 91%. In the classification of the normal and the minimal groups, the lateral temporal lobe did not increase the classification accuracy.

Hippocampal volume prediction studies

MRI volume studies also enable direct examination of the anatomic specificity of the prediction of reduced memory performance in normal and individuals and in the clinical decline to dementia in non-demented elderly individuals. In a recent longitudinal study, we observed that in elderly normal subjects (MMSE>27, $n=54$) the baseline volume of the hippocampus, but not the superior temporal gyrus, was related to delayed paragraph recall performance[112]. After a follow-up interval of 4 years, we observed in this same normal elderly cohort that the smaller baseline hippocampal volumes were predictive of disproportionately greater reductions in delayed recall performance[113]. Although the strength of this relationship was significant ($r=0.54$, $p<0.01$), the results were not sufficiently strong to provide clinically relevant predictions for individuals.

On the other hand, the volume data contribute to the prediction of future AD. Based on a very recent study, we now have preliminary evidence to indicate that, over 3 years, the volume reductions in baseline fusiform and middle inferior temporal lobe gyri predict the decline in MCI to AD with a very high degree of accuracy[114]. The baseline lateral temporal lobe volumes predicted who was going to decline to AD much more accurately than the medial temporal lobe alone and significantly added to it, reaching an overall diagnostic accuracy greater than 90%. These data indicate that the fusiform and middle–inferior temporal lobe gyri may be among the first temporal lobe neocortical sites affected in AD; atrophy in this area among non-demented individuals may herald the presence of future AD. Below we highlight some of our recent findings on the entorhinal cortex that appears to hold additional promise for the prognosis of decline among normal elderly individuals.

Relationship between hippocampal atrophy and memory in normal aging

We studied 126 of the elderly normal controls from the above cross-sectional study[115] in order to examine the relationship between hippocampal atrophy and neuropsychological test performance in normal aging. All the subjects selected for the study had MMSE scores of ≥28, indicating a very high level of functioning. All subjects underwent neuropsychological tests sensitive to performance differences in immediate and recent verbal recall. Of these subjects, 29% had hippocampal atrophy. With the psychometric measures used as a set of dependent variables in a multivariate design, with age and years of education as covariates, significant cognitive differences were observed between the groups positive and negative for hippocampal atrophy ($p<0.05$). *Post hoc* univariate comparisons demonstrated that the significant relationships were between hippocampal atrophy and the tests of delayed verbal memory ($p<0.01$) but not to the tests of immediate memory. This result is consistent with the pattern of memory dysfunction reported in subjects with circumscribed hippocampal lesions. To our knowledge, this was the first time these relationships were observed in normal elderly individuals. More recently, using hippocampal volumes in place of hippocampal atrophy[112], we replicated this hippocampus–delayed recall correlation in another normal elderly sample.

Entorhinal cortex studies

Anatomic validation of the MRI entorhinal cortex measurements

Using MRI, several attempts have been made to measure the volume of the entorhinal cortex in AD[116,117]. As the boundaries of the entorhinal and perirhinal cortices are poorly visible on MRI, the variability associated with the volume study probably accounts for the absence of reports of entorhinal cortex changes early in the course of AD. Recently, we published a method for estimating the surface area of the entorhinal cortex on MRI[118]. In order to validate our method, we used serial 3-mm sections stained with cresyl violet to define actual histological measures of entorhinal cortex volume and entorhinal cortex length as well as to estimate the cortical length using gyral landmarks visible both on the histological sections and on MRI. A total of 16 AD patients and four normal controls were studied. The true entorhinal cortex histological length was measured between the most medial boundary (pyriform cortex, or amygdala, or presubiculum, or parasubiculum, dependent on the rostrocaudal level)

and the most lateral points (referred to as perirhinal or transentorhinal cortex). Using the gyral landmarks, the measurements were made across all slices from the anterior end, defined as 3 mm posterior to the frontotemporal junction, to the posterior end, defined as the rostral pole of the lateral geniculate body. Across slices, the medial boundary of the entorhinal cortex was defined as the depth of the sulcus semianularis on anterior sections and the medial parahippocampal gyrus on posterior sections. The lateral boundary was the depth of the rhinal sulcus in anterior sections, and the depth of the collateral sulcus in the posterior sections (Figure 10). The lateral boundaries of the entorhinal cortex landmark lengths go beyond the entorhinal cortex histological lengths. Our studies show that this segment consists entirely of perirhinal cortex. The results showed a strong relationship between the volume of the entorhinal cortex and both the histology-based surface area ($r=0.94$, $p<0.001$) and the landmark-based surface area ($r=0.91$, $p<0.001$). The entorhinal measurements were significantly reduced in AD relative to normals ($p<0.01$) (volume 61%, histological surface area 49%, landmark length 45% and perirhinal surface area 44%).

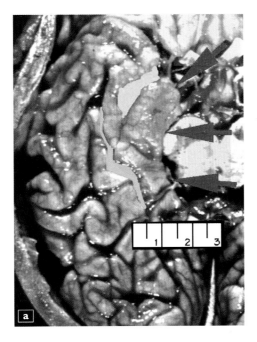 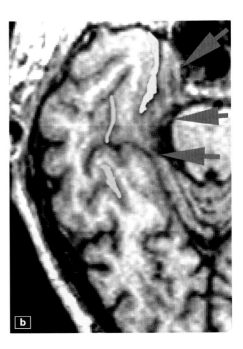

Figure 10 Ventral surface of the brain highlighting the medial surface of the entorhinal cortex (red arrows) and the rhinal (yellow) and collateral sulci (blue). (a) Postmortem specimen; (b) *in vivo* MRI

Entorhinal cortex atrophy, the diagnosis of AD and the relationship to hippocampal atrophy

After this validation study, the entorhinal cortex landmark measurement technique was applied to an *in vivo* sample, using a high-resolution MRI protocol. We obtained MRI scans for eight normal controls and eight patients with very mild AD matched for age, gender and education. The AD patients had MMSE scores of ≥24. For comparisons across brain regions, the entorhinal cortex surface area, the hippocampal volume and the superior temporal gyrus volumes were determined. Intracranial volumes, spanning the regions of interest, were determined by outlining the dural and tentorial margins and were used to correct for individual differences in head size. The entorhinal cortex landmark method differed by 27% between the normal and the AD groups ($p<0.001$). The hippocampal volumes differed by 12% ($p<0.05$) and the superior temporal gyrus volumes did not differ. In logistic regression models, the entorhinal cortex/head-size ratio correctly classified 100% of the controls and 87.5% of the AD patients ($p<0.001$), the hippocampal/head-size ratio classified 87.5% and 75% ($p<0.05$), and the superior temporal gyrus ratio classified 62.5% and 62.5% ($p<0.05$). In subsequent logistic regression models comparing the performance of the three variables, the entorhinal cortex/head-size ratio was consistently the superior predictor of group membership. Overall, these data indicated that a simple and anatomically valid MRI measurement of the surface area of the entorhinal cortex is potentially useful in the early diagnosis of AD. Moreover, these data suggest that, early in the course of AD, entorhinal cortex measurements may have superior diagnostic value over measurements of the hippocampus or the neocortex.

Conclusions

In vivo examination of the hippocampal region appears to be of descriptive value over the clinical course of AD. The data indicate that atrophic entorhinal and hippocampal changes appear early in the natural history of AD and are progressive. Atrophy of the hippocampus proper is relatively uncommon in normal elderly individuals. However, when such atrophic changes are present, they are associated with memory deficits. The data suggest that, in mildly impaired individuals, hippocampal atrophy appears to be related to the AD process as it predicts with high sensitivity and specificity the decline to AD levels of cognitive performance[91,104]. While the frequency of *in vivo* detected entorhinal cortex atrophy is currently unknown, entorhinal atrophy is more useful than hippocampal atrophy in differentiating normal elderly patients from age-matched patients with very early AD. These observations are in part supported by post-mortem studies that show increased numbers of NFTs and reduced numbers of neurons in the entorhinal cortex and hippocampus in both MCI patients[40] and normal elderly individuals[32].

In summary, it is universally observed at post-mortem examination that hippocampal atrophy occurs in AD. We now extend these observations by showing *in vivo* a remarkably high frequency of hippocampal atrophy among individuals with probable mild AD and MCI. The imaging data also show the consistent and necessary involvement of the lateral temporal lobe, particularly the fusiform and the middle–inferior gyri, in the statistical classification of AD patients relative to MCI patients. Perhaps, most importantly, the recent neuropathology and neuroimaging evidence points to an even earlier lesion that might be detected in the entorhinal cortex. Entorhinal cortex lesions may actually antedate the lesions of the hippocampus proper. Overall, these findings suggest that clinical capability might soon be reached for identification and measurement of brain changes in non-demented patients which place them at increased risk for memory decline, further brain damage and AD. It is anticipated that future therapeutic studies will probably use brain imaging measures, which are relatively free of education and cultural bias, for both study selection purposes and treatment outcome measures.

Acknowledgements

This work was made possible by grants from the National Institute on Aging: P30 AG08051, RO1 AG12101, AG13616, AG03051 and PO1 AG04220; and the New York State Office of Mental Retardation and Developmental Disabilities.

References

1. Schoenberg BS. Epidemiology of Alzheimer's disease and other dementing disorders. *J Chronic Dis* 1986;39:1095–104

2. Clark RF, Goate AM. Molecular genetics of Alzheimer's disease. *Arch Neurol* 1993;50:1164–72

3. Paykel ES, Brayne C, Huppert FA, *et al.* Incidence of dementia in a population older than 75 years in the United Kingdom. *Arch Gen Psychiat* 1994;51:325–32

4. Larrabee GJ, Crook TH. Estimated prevalence of age-associated memory impairment derived from standardized tests of memory function. *Int Psychogeriat* 1994;6:95–104

5. Braak H, Braak E. Neuropathological stageing of Alzheimer-related changes. *Acta Neuropathol* 1991;82:239–59

6. Giannakopoulos P, Hof PR, Mottier S, *et al.* Neuropathological changes in the cerebral cortex of 1258 cases from a geriatric hospital: retrospective clinicopathological evaluation of a 10-year autopsy population. *Acta Neuropathol* 1994; 87:456–68

7. Convit A, de Leon MJ, Tarshish C, *et al.* Specific hippocampal volume reductions in individuals at risk for Alzheimer's disease. *Neurobiol Aging* 1997;18:131–38

8. Amaral DG, Insausti R. Hippocampal formation. In Paxinos G, ed. *The Human Nervous System.* San Diego: Academic Press, 1990

9. Rosene DL, Van Hoesen GW. The hippocampal formation of the primate brain: a review of some comparative aspects of cytoarchitecture and connections. In Jones EG, Peters A, eds. *Cerebral Cortex,* vol. 6. New York: Plenum Press, 1987

10. Duvernoy HM. The human hippocampus. In *An Atlas of Applied Anatomy.* Munich: J.F. Bergmann Verlag, 1988

11. Convit A, McHugh PR, Wolf OT, *et al.* MRI volume of the amygdala: a reliable method allowing separation from the hippocampal formation. *Psychiatry Res Neuroimag* 1999; in press

12. Brodmann K. *Vergleichende lokalisationslehre der grosshirnrinde in ihren prinzipien dargestellt auf grund des zellenbaues.* Leipzig: Barth, 1909

13. Braak H. Zur pigmentoarchitektonic der Grosshirnrinde des Menschen. I. Regio entorhinalis. *Z Zellforsch* 1972;127:407–38

14. Vogt C, Vogt O. Allgemeinere Ergebnisse unserer Hirnforschung. *J Psychol Neurol* 1919;25:279–462

15. Rose M. Die sog, Riechrinde beim Menschen und beim Affem. II. Teil des 'Allocortex bei Tier und Mensch'. *J Psychol Neurol* 1927;34:261–401

16. Amaral DG, Insausti R, Cowan WM. The entorhinal cortex of the monkey: I. Cytoarchitectonic organization. *J Comp Neurol* 1987;264:326–55

17. Insausti R, Tunon T, Sobreviela T, *et al.* The human entorhinal cortex: a cytoarchitectonic analysis. *J Comp Neurol* 1995;355:171–98

18. Braak H. *Architectonics of the Human Telencephalic Cortex.* Berlin: Springer-Verlag, 1980

19. Suzuki WA, Amaral DG. Perirhinal and parahippocampal cortices of the macaque monkey: cortical afferents. *J Comp Neurol* 1994;350:497–533

20. Van Hoesen GW. The parahippocamal gyrus: new observations regarding its cortical connections in the monkey. *TINS* 1982;345–50

21. Insausti R, Amaral DG, Cowan WM. The entorhinal cortex of the monkey: III. Subcortical afferents. *J Comp Neurol* 1987;264:396–408

22. Witter MP, Amaral DG. Entorhinal cortex of the monkey: V. Projections to the dentate gyrus, hippocampus, and subicular complex. *J Comp Neurol* 1991;307:437–59

23. Reisberg B, Ferris SH, de Leon MJ, Crook T. The global deterioration scale for assessment of primary degenerative dementia. *Am J Psychiat* 1982;139:1136–9

24. Hyman BT, Van Hoesen GW, Damasio AR, Barnes CL. Alzheimer's disease: cell-specific pathology isolates the hippocampal formation. *Science* 1984;225:1168–70

25. Ball MJ, Hachinski V, Fox A, *et al*. A new definition of Alzheimer's disease: a hippocampal dementia. *Lancet* 1985;1:14–16

26. Bobinski M, Wegiel J, Tarnawski M, *et al*. Relationships between regional neuronal loss and neurofibrillary changes in the hippocampal formation and duration and severity of Alzheimer disease. *J Neuropathol Exp Neurol* 1997;56:414–20

27. Bobinski MJ, Wegiel J, Wisniewski HM, *et al*. Neurofibrillary pathology – correlation with hippocampal formation atrophy in Alzheimer disease. *Neurobiol Aging* 1996;17:909–19

28. Davies DC, Horwood N, Isaacs SL, Mann DMA. The effect of age and Alzheimer's disease on pyramidal neuron density in the individual fields of the hippocampal formation. *Acta Neuropathol* 1992;83:510–17

29. Bouras C, Hof PR, Giannakopoulos P, *et al*. Regional distribution of neurofibrillary tangles and senile plaques in the cerebral cortex of elderly patients: a quantitative evaluation of a one-year autopsy population from a geriatric hospital. *Cereb Cortex* 1994;4:138–50

30. Bobinski M, Wegiel J, Wisniewski HM, *et al*. Atrophy of hippocampal formation subdivisions correlates with stage and duration of Alzheimer disease. *Dementia* 1995;6:205–10

31. Reisberg B. Functional assessment staging (FAST). *Psychopharmacol Bull* 1988;24:653–9

32. Gomez-Isla T, Price JL, McKeel DW Jr, *et al*. Profound loss of layer II entorhinal cortex neurons occurs in very mild Alzheimer's disease. *J Neurosci* 1996;16:4491–500

33. West MJ, Coleman PD, Flood DG, Troncoso JC. Differences in the pattern of hippocampal neuronal loss in normal ageing and Alzheimer's disease. *Lancet* 1994;344:769–72

34. Hof PR, Bierer LM, Perl DP, *et al*. Evidence for early vulnerability of the medial and inferior aspects of the temporal lobe in an 82-year-old patient with preclinical signs of dementia: regional and laminar distribution of neurofibrillary tangles and senile plaques. *Arch Neurol* 1992;49:946–53

35. Hirano A, Zimmerman HM. Alzheimer's neurofibrillary changes. *Arch Neurol* 1962;7:227–42

36. Kemper TL. Senile dementia: a focal disease in the temporal lobe. In Nandy E, ed. *Senile Dementia: A Biomedical Approach*. New York: Elsevier, 1978

37. Mann DMA, Esiri MM. The pattern of acquisition of plaques and tangles in the brains of patients under 50 years of age with Down syndrome. *J Neurol Sci* 1989;89:169–79

38. Arriagada PV, Marzloff K, Hyman BT. Distribution of Alzheimer-type pathologic changes in nondemented elderly individuals matches the pattern in Alzheimer's disease. *Neurology* 1992;42:1681–8

39. Langui D, Probst A, Ulrich J. Alzheimer's changes in non-demented and demented patients: a statistical approach to their relationships. *Acta Neuropathol* 1995;89:57–62

40. Price JL, Davis PB, Morris JC, White DL. The distribution of tangles, plaques and related immunohistochemical markers in healthy aging and Alzheimer's disease. *Neurobiol Aging* 1991;12:295–312

41. Morris JC, McKeel DW, Storandt M, *et al*. Very mild Alzheimer's disease: informant-based clinical, psychometric, and pathological distinction from normal aging. *Neurology* 1991;41:469–78

42. de la Monte SM. Quantitation of cerebral atrophy in preclinical and end-stage Alzheimer's disease. *Ann Neurol* 1989;25:450–9

43. Braak H, Braak E, Yilmazer D, Bohl J. Functional anatomy of human hippocampal formation and related structures. *J Child Neurol* 1996;11:265–75

44. Insausti R, Amaral DG, Cowan WM. The entorhinal cortex of the monkey: II. Cortical afferents. *J Comp Neurol* 1987;264:356–95

45. Nakamura K, Kubota K. The primate temporal pole: its putative role in object recognition and memory. *Behav Brain Res* 1996;77:53–77

46. Squire LR. Memory and the hippocampus: a synthesis from findings with rats, monkeys, and humans. *Psychol Rev* 1992;99:195–231

47. Pickering-Brown SM, Mann DMA, Bourke JP, *et al.* Apolipoprotein E4 and Alzheimer's disease pathology in Lewy body disease and in other β-amyloid-forming diseases. *Lancet* 1994;343:1155

48. Higuchi S-I, Miyashita Y. Formation of mnemonic neuronal responses to visual paired associates in inferotemporal cortex is impaired by perirhinal and entorhinal lesions. *Proc Natl Acad Sci USA* 1996;93:739–43

49. Miyashita Y. Interior temporal cortex: where visual perception meets memory. *Ann Rev Neurosci* 1993;16:245–63

50. Zola-Morgan S, Squire LR, Ramus SJ. Severity of memory impairment in monkeys as a function of locus and extent of damage within the medial temporal lobe memory system. *Hippocampus* 1994;4:483–95

51. Horel JA. The neuroanatomy of amnesia. A critique of the hippocampal memory hypothesis. *Brain* 1978;101:403–45

52. Murray EA, Mishkin M. Visual recognition in monkeys following rhinal cortical ablations combined with either amygdalectomy or hippocampectomy. *J Neurosci* 1986;6:1991–2003

53. Suzuki WA, Zola-Morgan S, Squire LR, Amaral DG. Lesions of the perirhinal and parahippocampal cortices in the monkey produce long-lasting memory impairment in the visual and tactual modalities. *J Neurosci* 1993;13:2430–51

54. Zola-Morgan S, Squire LR, Amaral DG, Suzuki WA. Lesions of perirhinal and parahippocampal cortex that spare the amygdala and hippocampal formation produce severe memory impairment. *J Neurosci* 1989;9:4355–70

55. Fahy FL, Riches IP, Brown MW. Neuronal activity related to visual recognition memory: long-term memory and the encoding of recency and familiarity information in the primate anterior and medial inferior temporal and rhinal cortex. *Exp Brain Res* 1993;96:457–72

56. Meunier M, Bachevalier J, Mishkin M, Murray EA. Effects on visual recognition of combined and separate ablations of the entorhinal and perirhinal cortex in rhesus monkeys. *J Neurosci* 1993;13:5418–32

57. Suzuki WA. The anatomy, physiology and functions of the perirhinal cortex. *Curr Opin Neurobiol* 1996;6:179–86

58. Leonard BW, Amaral DG, Squire LR, Zola-Morgan S. Transient memory impaiment in monkeys with bilateral lesions of the entorhinal cortex. *J Neurosci* 1995;15:5637–59

59. Liu P, Bilkey DK. Direct connection between perirhinal cortex and hippocampus is a major constituent of the lateral perforant path. *Hippocampus* 1996;6:125–34

60. Mizutani T, Kasahara M. Degeneration of the intrahippocampal routes of the perforant and alvear pathways in senile dementia of Alzheimer type. *Neurosci Lett* 1995;184:141–4

61. Poduri A, Beason-Held LL, Moss MB, *et al.* CA3 neuronal degeneration follows chronic entorhinal cortex lessions. *Neurosci Lett* 1995;197:1–4

62. Mizutani T, Kasahara M. Hippocampal atrophy secondary to entorhinal cortical degeneration in Alzheimer-type dementia. *Neurosci Lett* 1997;222:119–22

63. Ueki A, Miwa C, Oohara K, Miyoshi K. Histological evidence for cholinergic alteration in the hippocampus following entorhinal cortex lesion. *J Neurol Sci* 1996;142:7–11

64. Craik FIM, Jennings JM. Human memory. In Craik FIM, Salthouse TA, eds. *The Handbook of Aging and Cognition.* Hillsdale, NJ: Lawrence Erlbaum Associates, 1992

65. Flicker C, Ferris SH, Crook T, *et al.* Cognitive decline in advanced age: future directions for the psychometric differentiation of normal and pathological age changes in cognitive function. *Dev Neuropsychol* 1986;2:309–22

66. Hartley AA. Attention. In Craik FIM, Salthouse TA, eds. *The Handbook of Aging and Cognition.* Hillsdale NJ; Lawrence Erlbaum Associates, 1992

67. Salthouse TA. Reasoning and spatial abilities. In Craik FIM, Salthouse TA, eds. *The Handbook of Aging and Cognition.* Hillsdale, NJ: Lawrence Erlbaum Associates, 1992

68. Ivnik RJ, Malec JF, Tangalos EG, *et al.* The Auditory–Verbal Learning Test (AVLT): norms for ages 55 years and older. Psychological assessment. *J Consult Clin Psychol* 1990;2:304–12

69. Botwinick J, Siegler HC. Intellectual ability among the elderly: simultaneous cross-sectional and longitudinal comparisons. *Dev Psychol* 1980; 16:49–53

70. Hultsch DF, Hertzog C, Small BJ, *et al.* Short-term longitudinal change in cognitive performance in later life. *Psychol Aging* 1992;7:571–84

71. Lachman ME. Perceptions of intellectual aging: antecedent or consequence of intellectual functioning? *Dev Psychol* 1983;19:482–98

72. McCarty SM, Siegler IC, Logue PE. Cross-sectional and longitudinal patterns of three wechsler memory scale subtests. *J Gerontol* 1982;37:169–75

73. Mitrushina M, Satz P. Changes in cognitive functioning associated with normal aging. *Arch Clin Neuropsychol* 1991;6:49–60

74. Rinn WE. Mental decline in normal aging: a review. *J Geriat Psychiat Neurol* 1988;1:144–58

75. Colsher PL, Wallace RB. Longitudinal application of cognitive function measures in a defined population of community-dwelling elders. *Ann Epidemiol* 1991;1:215–30

76. Bondi MW, Monsh AU, Galasko D, *et al.* Preclinical cognitive markers of dementia of the Alzheimer type. *Neuropsychology* 1994;8:374–84

77. Hanninen T, Hallikainen M, Koivisto K, *et al.* A follow-up study of age-associated memory impairment: neuropsychological predictors of dementia. *J Am Geriatr Sci* 1995;43:1007–15

78. Kluger A, Ferris SH. Scales for the assessment of Alzheimer's disease. In Davidson M, ed. *The Psychiatric Clinics of North America: Alzheimer's Disease.* Philadelphia: W. B. Saunders, 1991

79. Neary D, Snowden JS, Bowen DM, *et al.* Neuropsychological syndromes in presenile dementia due to cerebral atrophy. *J Neurol Neurosurg Psychiatry* 1986;49:163–74

80. Petersen RC, Smith G, Kokmen E, *et al.* Memory function in normal aging. *Neurology* 1992; 42:396–401

81. Sim A, Sussman I. Alzheimer's disease: its natural history and differential diagnosis. *J Nerv Ment Dis* 1962;135:489–99

82. Tierney MC, Szalai JP, Snow WG, *et al.* Prediction of probable Alzheimer's disease in memory-impaired patients: a prospective longitudinal study. *Neurology* 1996;46:661–5

83. Welsh K, Butters N, Hughes J, *et al.* Detection of abnormal memory decline in mild cases of Alzheimer's disease using CERAD neuropsychological measures. *Arch Neurol* 1991;48:278–81

84. Flicker C, Ferris SH, Reisberg B. Mild cognitive impairment in the elderly: predictors of dementia. *Neurology* 1991;41:1006–9

85. Fuld PA, David MM, Blau AD, *et al.* Object-memory evaluation for prospective detection of dementia in normal functioning elderly: predictive and normative data. *J Clin Exp Neuropsychol* 1990;12:520–8

86. Masur DM, Fuld PA, Blau AD, *et al.* Predicting development of dementia in the elderly with the selective reminding test. *J Clin Exp Neuropsychol* 1990;12:529–38

87. Masur DM, Sliwinski M, Lipton RB, *et al.* Neuropsychological prediction of dementia and the absence of dementia in healthy elderly persons. *Neurology* 1994;44:1427–32

88. Weingartner HJ, Kawas C, Rawlings R, Shapiro M. Changes in semantic memory in early stage Alzheimer's disease patients. *Gerontologist* 1993;33:637–43

89. Mesulam MM. Large-scale neurocognitive networks and distributed processing for attention, language, and memory. *Neurol Prog* 1990;28:597–613

90. de Leon MJ, George AE, Ferris SH, *et al.* Positron emission tomography and computed tomography assessments of the aging human brain. *J Comput Assist Tomogr* 1984;8:88–94

91. de Leon MJ, George AE, Stylopoulos LA, *et al.* Early marker for Alzheimer's disease: the atrophic hippocampus. *Lancet* 1989;2:672–3

92. de Leon MJ, McRae T, Tsai JR, *et al.* Abnormal cortisol response in Alzheimer's disease linked to hippocampal atrophy. *Lancet* 1988;2:391–2

93. Kesslak JP, Nalcioglu O, Cotman CW. Quantification of magnetic resonance scans for hippocampal and parahippocampal atrophy in Alzheimer's disease. *Neurology* 1991;41:51–4

94. Press GA, Amaral DG, Squire LR. Hippocampal abnormalities in amnesic patients revealed by high-resolution magnetic resonance imaging. *Nature* 1989;341:54–7

95. Seab JP, Jagust WS, Wong SFS, *et al.* Quantitative NMR measurements of hippocampal atrophy in Alzheimer's disease. *Magnet Reson Med* 1988; 8:200–8

96. Convit A, de Leon MJ, Golomb J, *et al.* Hippocampal atrophy in early Alzheimer's disease: anatomic specificity and validation. *Psychiatr Q* 1993;64:371–87

97. Convit A, de Leon MJ, Tarshish C, *et al.* Hippocampal volume losses in minimally impaired elderly. *Lancet* 1995;345:266

98. Deweer B, Lehericy S, Pillon B, *et al.* Memory disorders in probable Alzheimer's disease: the role of hippocampal atrophy as shown with MRI. *J Neurol Neurosurg Psychiatry* 1995;58:590–7

99. Ikeda M, Tanabe H, Nakagawa Y, *et al.* MRI-based quantitative assessment of the hippocampal region in very mild to moderate Alzheimer's disease. *Neuroradiology* 1994;36:7–10

100. Jack CR, Petersen RC, O'Brien PC, Tangalos EG. MR-based hippocampal volumetry in the diagnosis of Alzheimer's disease. *Neurology* 1992;42:183–8

101. Jernigan TL, Salmon DP, Butters N, Hesselink JR. Cerebral structure on MRI, Part II: specific changes in Alzheimer's and Huntington's diseases. *Biol Psychiatry* 1991;29:68–81

102. Lehericy S, Baulac M, Chiras J, *et al.* Amygdalohippocampal MR volume measurements in the early stages of Alzheimer disease. *Am J Neuroradiol* 1994;15:929–37

103. de Leon MJ, George AE, Golomb J, *et al.* Frequency of hippocampus atrophy in normal elderly and Alzheimer's disease patients. *Neurobiol Aging* 1997;18:1–11

104. de Leon MJ, Golomb J, George AE, *et al.* The radiologic prediction of Alzheimer's disease: the atrophic hippocampal formation. *Am J Neuroradiol* 1993;14:897–906

105. Jobst KA, Smith AD, Szatmari M, *et al.* Rapidly progressing atrophy of medial temporal lobe in Alzheimer's disease. *Lancet* 1994;343:829–30

106. Scheltens P, Leys D, Barkhof F, *et al.* Atrophy of medial temporal lobes on MRI in 'probable' Alzheimer's disease and normal aging: diagnostic value and neuropsychological correlates. *J Neurol Neurosurg Psychiatry* 1992;55:967–72

107. Stout JC, Jernigan TL, Archibald SL, Salmon DP. Association of dementia severity with cortical gray matter and abnormal white matter volumes in dementia of Alzheimer type. *Arch Neurol* 1996;53:742–9

108. Aylward EH, Rasmusson DX, Brandt J, *et al.* CT measurement of suprasellar cistern predicts rate of cognitive decline in Alzheimer's disease. *J Int Neuropsychol Soc* 1996;2:89–95

109. de Leon MJ, George AE, Convit A, *et al.* MR measurement of the medial temporal lobe changes in Alzheimer disease: the case for the interuncal distance. *Am J Neuroradiol* 1994;15:1286–90

110. Folstein MF, Folstein SE, McHugh PR. Mini-mental state: a practical method for grading the cognitive state of patients for the clinician. *J Psychiat Res* 1975;12:189–98

111. de Leon MJ. Neuroimaging and the early diagnosis of Alzheimer disease. *6th International Conference on Alzheimer's Disease and Related Disorders,* 1998, Amsterdam

112. Golomb J, Kluger A, de Leon MJ, *et al.* Hippocampal formation size in normal human aging: a correlate of delayed secondary memory performance. *Learning Memory* 1994;1:45–54

113. Golomb J, Kluger A, de Leon MJ, *et al.* Hippocampal formation size predicts declining memory performance in normal aging. *Neurology* 1996;47:810–13

114. Convit A, de Asis J, de Leon MJ, *et al.* The fusiform gyrus as the first neocortical site in Alzheimer's disease. *6th International Conference on Alzheimer's Disease and Related Disorders,* 1998, Amsterdam

115. Golomb J, de Leon MJ, Kluger A, *et al.* Hippocampal atrophy in normal aging: an association with recent memory impairment. *Arch Neurol* 1993;50:967–73

116. Juottonen K, Laakso MP, Insausti R, *et al.* Volumes of the entorhinal and perirhinal cortices in Alzheimer's Disease. *Neurobiol Aging* 1998;19:15–22

117. Pearlson GD, Harris GJ, Powers RE, *et al.* Quantitative changes in mesial temporal volume, regional cerebral blood flow, and cognition in Alzheimer's disease. *Arch Gen Psychiat* 1992;49:402–8

118. Bobinski M, de Leon MJ, Convit A, *et al.* MRI of entorhinal cortex in mild Alzheimer's disease. *Lancet* 1999;353:38–40

5 Neuropathological stages of Alzheimer's disease

Heiko Braak and Eva Braak

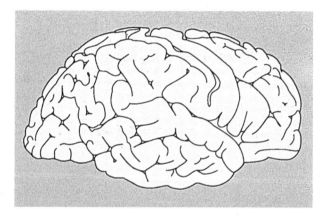

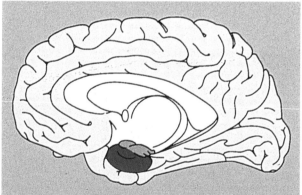

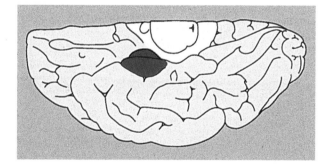

The insidious onset of Alzheimer`s disease (AD) is characterized by a subtle decline of memory function in a state of clear consciousness. As time passes, changes in personality, deterioration of verbal communication, impairment in visuospatial tasks and, eventually, dysfunction of the motor system are gradually added to the initial symptoms. This steady aggravation of symptoms reflects the gradual expansion of AD-related brain destruction, which begins in specific limbic areas of the cortex and then spreads, in a predictable pattern, across the hippocampus to the neocortex and a number of subcortical nuclei. This sequence of lesion progression and development may be more easily understood if the major neural connections of the structures involved are briefly reviewed[1,2].

The telencephalic cortex consists of two basic types of gray matter: neocortex and allocortex (Figure 1). The small allocortex is located primarily in the anteromedial portions of the temporal lobe and includes limbic system centers such as the hippocampal formation, presubiculum and entorhinal region. The subcortical amygdala is closely related.

Figure 1 The cerebral cortex consists of two basic types of gray matter: the extensive homogeneous neocortex (yellow), and the small heterogeneous allocortex. The allocortex is located chiefly in the anteromedial portions of the temporal lobe, and includes limbic system centers such as the hippocampal formation (orange), presubiculum and entorhinal region (red). The subcortical amygdala is closely related

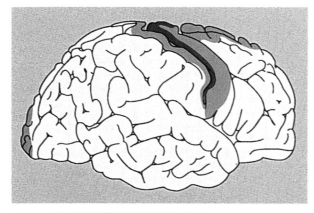

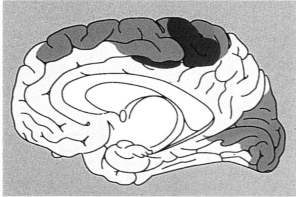

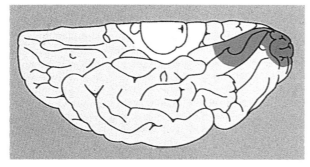

Figure 2 The neocortex is particularly extensive in the human brain. The frontal, parietal, occipital and temporal neocortices each comprises a primary core field (blue or red areas), a secondary belt region (green or orange areas) and related higher-order processing areas (yellow), often referred to as 'association areas'

The neocortex is particularly extensive in the human brain. In the frontal, parietal, occipital and temporal regions, the neocortex comprises a primary core field and a belt region, and related higher-order processing areas (association areas; Figure 2).

Normally, somatosensory, visual and auditory data proceed through the core and belt fields to

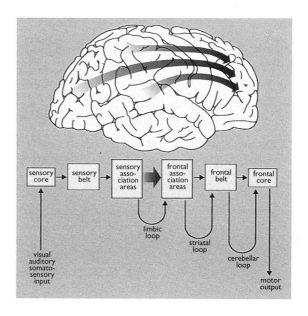

Figure 3 Somatosensory, visual and auditory information proceeds through the respective neocortical core and belt fields to a variety of related association areas. From there, data are transported *via* long corticocortical pathways to the prefrontal cortex. Tracts generated from this highest organizational level of the brain guide the information back *via* the striatal and cerebellar loops to the primary motor field. Reproduced from reference 2, with permission

the related association areas from which the data are conveyed, *via* long corticocortical feed-forward pathways, to the prefrontal cortex. Tracts generated in this highest organizational level of the brain then transmit the information, *via* the frontal belt (premotor areas), to the primary motor field. Minor routes are corticocortical feedback projections. The striatal loop and the cerebellar loop provide the major routes for this data transfer and, thus, the basal ganglia, many of the nuclei of the lower brain stem and the cerebellum are incorporated into the regulation of cortical output.

In addition to this system of short and long projections from the neocortical sensory association areas to the prefrontal cortex, there is also an orderly sequence of corticocortical connections which eventually converges upon the entorhinal region (port of entry: transentorhinal region) and the amygdala (port of entry: lateral nucleus). Neo-

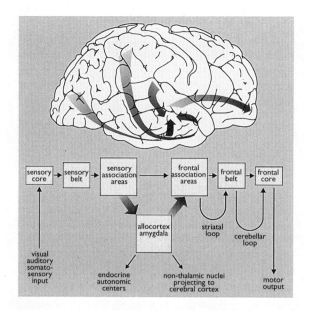

Figure 4 Part of this stream of data running from the sensory association areas to the prefrontal cortex branches off to eventually converge upon the entorhinal region and amygdala (afferent leg of the limbic loop). Projections from the entorhinal region, amygdala and hippocampal formation (efferent leg of the limbic loop) exert an influence upon the prefrontal cortex. Reproduced from reference 2, with permission

cortical information thus provides the most important input to the human limbic system (Figures 3 and 4).

Many of the allocortical structures that process neocortical data are a late development both phylogenetically and ontogenetically. In particular, the transentorhinal region increases markedly in size going up the primate ladder. It is, for the most part, hidden in the depths of the rhinal sulcus and accompanies the entorhinal region, which extends over the anterior portions of the parahippocampal gyrus.

In addition to neocortical information, the human entorhinal region receives a strong input from the basolateral nuclei of the amygdala and from centers of limbic circuits *via* the presubiculum; projections from olfactory areas are sparse and rudimentary. The entorhinal cortex exhibits a complex lamination pattern. The superficial cellular layer with its con-

spicuous islands of multipolar projection cells and subjacent layers of the outer main stratum generate the perforant path through which neocortical and limbic data are transferred to the hippocampal formation. A dense feedback projection from the hippocampus runs *via* a deep entorhinal layer to the neocortex.

The development of an upright gait freed the upper limbs from their usual tasks and allowed them to become flexible, less specialized, organs capable of further development. Similarly, the reduction in olfactory ability probably freed the entorhinal cortex and rendered internal reorganization possible. The entorhinal region in higher primates and humans functions predominantly as an interface between the neocortex and the limbic system.

Projections from the hippocampal formation, entorhinal region, and amygdala contribute to the efferent leg of the limbic loop. Many of these efferents terminate in the ventral 'limbic' striatum. The data are then transferred *via* the ventral pallidum and mediodorsal thalamic nucleus to the prefrontal cortex. In addition, the amygdala sends dense projections to all non-thalamic nuclei, which project diffusely upon the cerebral cortex and include the cholinergic nuclei of the basal forebrain, histaminergic tuberomamillary nucleus of the hypothalamus, dopaminergic nuclei of the ventral tegmentum, serotonergic anterior raphe nuclei and noradrenergic locus ceruleus. The amygdala is also the chief organ involved in processing viscerosensory information and is the control central for visceromotor functions.

The components of the limbic loop thus receive a broad range of afferents which serve to integrate somatosensory, auditory and visual exteroceptive data with interoceptive stimuli from the nuclei that process viscerosensory data. These limbic loop components generate projections which not only exert an influence on the highest organizational component of the human brain – the prefrontal cortex – but also guide the visceromotor and endocrine centers. Thus, the limbic loop is considered to be important not only for the maintenance of emo-

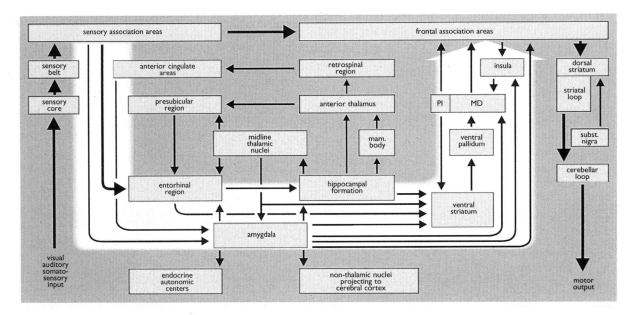

Figure 5 The limbic loop: The large white arrow emphasizes its strategic position between the neocortical sensory association areas and the prefrontal cortex. The hippocampal formation, entorhinal region and amygdala are densely interconnected and, together, the three represent the highest organizational level of the limbic system. cerebell loop, cerebellar loop; mam body, mamillary body; MD, mediodorsal thalamic nuclei; Pf, parafascicular nucleus; striat loop, striatal loop; subst nigra, substantia nigra. Reproduced from reference 2, with permission

tional stability, learning ability and memory function, but also for the regulation of endocrine and autonomic functions. It is precisely these areas that are particularly susceptible to grave pathological changes in AD[1,3,4] (Figure 5).

The destructive process underlying AD exhibits a characteristic area-specific, lamina-specific and even cell-type-specific distribution pattern[3]. Most conspicuous is the progressive deposition of virtually insoluble abnormal proteins, both between and within the nerve cells[5]. The extracellular deposits consist mainly of β-amyloid protein whereas abnormally phosphorylated tau protein contributes to the formation of the intraneuronal changes. Tau protein normally stabilizes the microtubules of the neuronal cytoskeleton. A variety of other substances accompany both the β-amyloid deposits and abnormal tau protein.

Amyloid deposits

The hydrophobic self-aggregating β-amyloid protein precipitates to plaque-like deposits which appear gradually at specific sites of predilection.

Inconspicuous, but extensive, cloud-like amyloid deposits with blurred boundaries are formed transiently in some deep cortical layers. The white substance and fiber tracts that run through amyloid-laden gray matter (fornix, mamillothalamic tract, anterior commissure) only occasionally show precipitations. The perforant path, in contrast, is replete with amyloid deposits. Sharply outlined globular plaques of variable diameter represent the more stable and mature forms of amyloid deposition. However, the local changes in the extracellular milieu which initiate the precipitation of amyloid remains unknown.

An inverse relationship is observed between the degree of myelination and the density of amyloid deposition in cortical layers and areas. Portions of the cortex dominated by pyramidal cells rich in lipofuscin granules also show denser accumulations of amyloid deposits than those areas and layers with sparsely pigmented neurons. Proliferation of the amyloid deposits is mediated by many as yet undetermined processes. The number of deposits increases until a certain level of density is reached. Yet, even at maximum density, a consid-

Figure 6 Hydrophobic self-aggregating amyloid protein precipitates to plaque-like deposits which appear gradually at specific predilection sites. Three stages in the gradual evolution of cortical amyloid precipitation are distinguished. Initially, deposition occurs in the poorly myelinated areas of the basal temporal neocortex, mostly in the form of diffuse plaques in layers III and V (stage A)

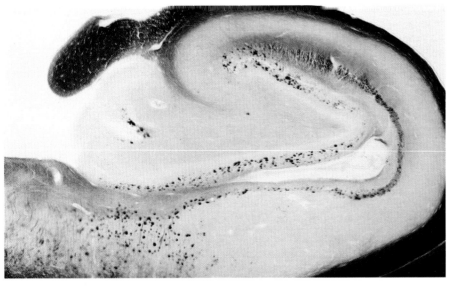

Figure 7 The perforant path becomes densely festooned with amyloid deposits as it pierces the subiculum and extends through the molecular layers of the CA1 sector and fascia dentata (stage B). In contrast, the white substance and other fiber tracts which traverse the amyloid-laden gray matter (fornix, mamillothalamic tract, anterior commissure) only occasionally show amyloid deposition

erable amount of the gray matter remains devoid of amyloid precipitations.

Three stages in the gradual evolution of cortical precipitations can be distinguished[3]. Deposition is first seen in the poorly myelinated areas of the basal temporal neocortex (stage A; Figure 6). From there, the alterations spread to adjoining neocortical areas, initially sparing the belt regions and primary fields. The perforant path then becomes studded with deposits as it extends through the hippocampal formation (stage B; Figures 7 and 8). The end

stage exhibits deposits in virtually all cortical areas, including the densely myelinated primary areas of the neocortex (stage C; Figures 9–12). Many individuals exhibit no amyloid deposition, even at a very advanced age whereas others, in contrast, develop the abnormal protein early in life[6] (Figure 13).

The term 'amyloid angiopathy' refers to amyloid precipitations in close connection to the abluminal basement membrane of the cerebral vessels. The predilection sites of these changes differ from those of the spherical amyloid deposits. A severe degree of amyloid angiopathy may be seen with no spherical cortical deposition and *vice versa*.

Figure 8 Spherical amyloid deposits in the basal temporal neocortex rapidly increase in number and, gradually, are then found in the adjoining neocortical association areas, at first sparing the more richly myelinated belt regions and primary areas of the neocortex (stage B). At this stage, the hippocampal formation and entorhinal region are still devoid of, or only mildly involved with, amyloid deposition

Figure 9 End-stage amyloid precipitation results in deposits in virtually all cortical areas, including the densely myelinated primary areas of the neocortex (stage C). In the primary visual field (striate area) shown here, the myelin-rich zone (line of Gennari) displays pale-staining amyloid deposits

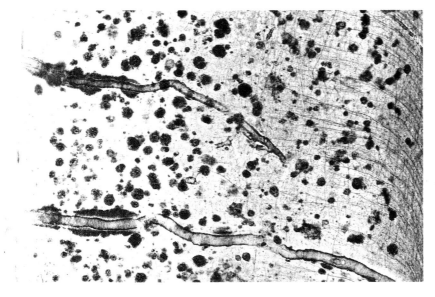

Figure 10 The term 'amyloid (congophilic) angiopathy' refers to amyloid precipitation in close connection to the abluminal basement membrane of small vessels in the leptomeninges and subjacent brain tissue. Even at end-stage C (shown here), however, a considerable amount of gray matter remains devoid of amyloid deposition

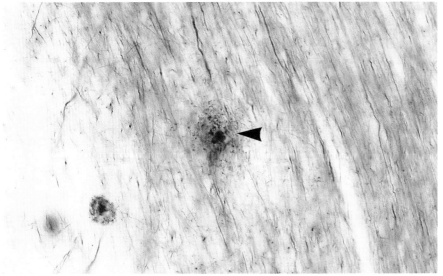

Figure 11 Initially, pale-staining amyloid strands are seen in the deep cortical layers and subjacent white matter. Eventually, the amyloid condenses into tightly packed granules surrounded by diffuse precipitations of decreasing intensity from the center to the periphery (white matter plaque; arrow). There is no relationship between the depth of amyloid infiltration into the white substance and the duration of the disease

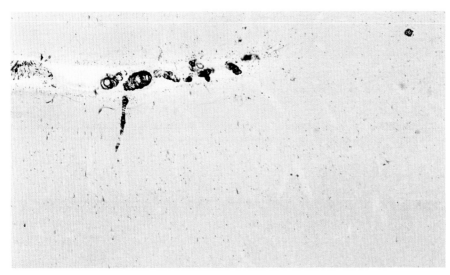

Figure 12 Predilection sites of amyloid (congophilic) angiopathy differ from those of spherical amyloid deposition in cortical gray matter. In specific patients, there may be amyloid angiopathy without spherical cortical amyloid deposits (as shown here) and *vice versa*

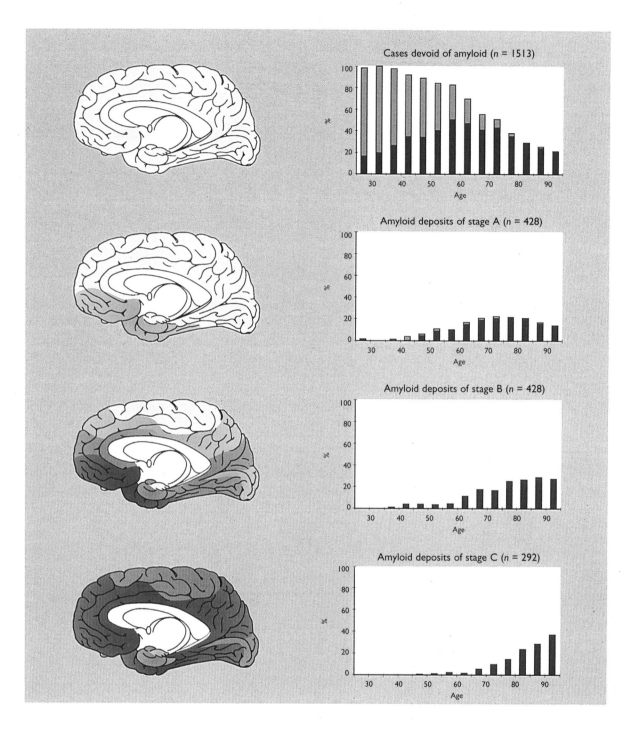

Figure 13 Pattern of distribution of amyloid deposits in the course of AD (left). In stage A, initial deposition is in the basal neocortex. In stage B, deposits occur in virtually all neocortical association areas whereas the hippocampal formation remains only mildly involved. In stage C, deposition extends throughout the entire cerebral cortex. The increasing color intensity reflects the growing density of deposition. The graphs show the frequency of amyloid stages in 2661 non-selected autopsy cases (right) in relation to age, with one subgroup devoid of neurofibrillary changes (light blue) and another expressing neurofibrillary changes regardless of stage (I–VI; dark blue). Reproduced from reference 6, with permission

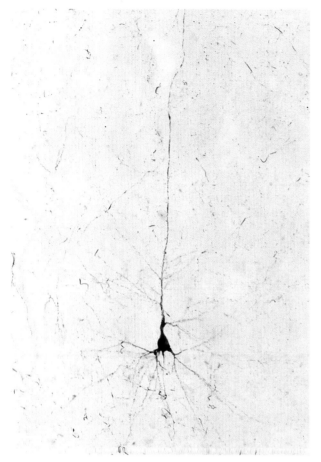

Figure 14 Histological section showing deposition of abnormally phosphorylated tau protein in a nerve cell

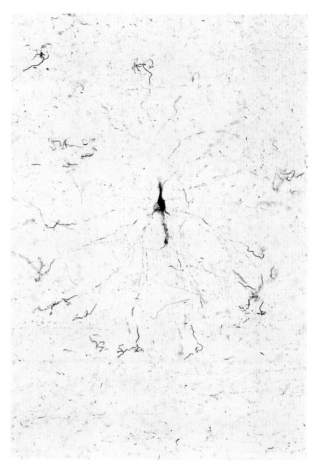

Figure 15 Histological section showing damage to the dendrites of a nerve cell containing abnormal tau protein

Neurofibrillary changes

The most outstanding pathological feature of AD is the progressive deposition of abnormally phosphorylated tau protein in a few susceptible types of nerve cells[7,8]. Specific antibodies that react with the abnormal tau protein (AT8) allow visualization of the altered cells with all their neurites. Specific projection cells of the transentorhinal region (Figure 14) are the first cortical neurons to show the changes. Initially, the AT8-immunoreactive neurons exhibit no obvious destruction of their neurites. Aggregation to a solid argyrophilic neurofibrillary tangle has not yet taken place[8].

Sooner or later, destruction of the nerve cell processes becomes apparent. The most conspicuous change is in the distal segments of the dendrites, which follow a curved and tortuous course and exhibit many varicosities and short appendages. With this degree of destruction, slender argyrophilic neuropil threads appear within the altered distal dendrites and, shortly thereafter, the formation of a neurofibrillary tangle begins in the soma[8] (Figures 15 and 16).

The intraneuronal material is generally deposited symmetrically in both hemispheres in the form of neurofibrillary tangles (NFTs), neuropil threads (NTs) and argyrophilic components of neuritic plaques (NPs). The first changes to occur are generally in the form of NTs and NFTs; NPs develop later. NFTs develop within the somata of nerve cells and often adopt the shape of the parent cell body. Slender NTs are found in the distal dendrites of tangle-bearing nerve cells. Spherical NPs consist of distended argyrophilic neurites filled with abnormal tau protein, dystrophic non-argyrophilic neu-

65

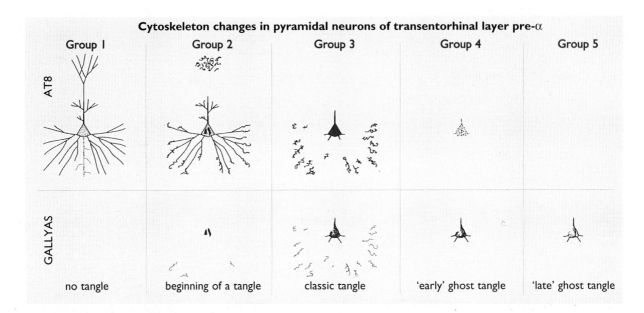

Figure 16 Progression of AD-related changes of the neuronal cytoskeleton in susceptible cortical pyramidal cells. Sequential changes in AT8-immunoreaction compared with a corresponding pattern in Gallyas silver-stained sections demonstrate the development of neurofibrillary changes. Reproduced from reference 8, with permission

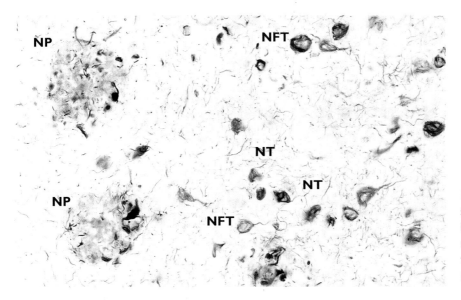

Figure 17 Histological section showing the three forms taken by abnormal intraneuronal material. NFT, neurofibrillary tangle; NT, neuropil thread; NP, neuritic plaque

rites, changed astrocytes and microglial cells. Amyloid is generally present in the form of a compact core and peripheral infiltration (Figures 17–19).

These abnormalities of the neuronal cytoskeleton develop slowly over time and undergo remarkable structural changes as they appear, grow to maturity and eventually disappear from the tissue[3,4,7–9]. Many individuals remain devoid of these altera-

tions or develop only the initial changes at a very advanced age whereas others may present with lesions surprisingly early in life. There is a continuum of changes, starting with the first NFT and extending to the intense degree of intraneuronal changes seen in fully developed AD.

Only a small number of the many different types of neurons in the brain are prone to develop these

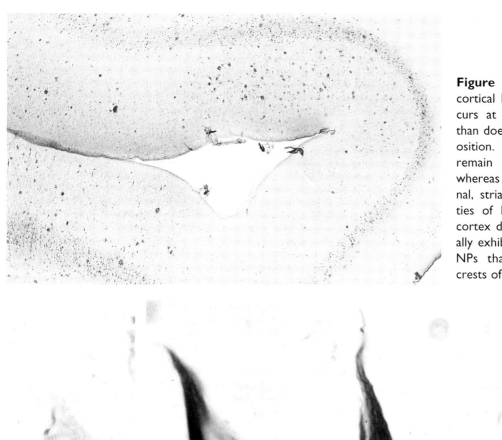

Figure 18 The distribution of cortical NPs is patchy, and occurs at much lower densities than does amyloid protein deposition. A few cortical areas remain virtually free of NPs whereas other areas (ectorhinal, striate) exhibit high densities of NP development. The cortex deep in the sulci generally exhibits a higher density of NPs than that covering the crests of the gyri

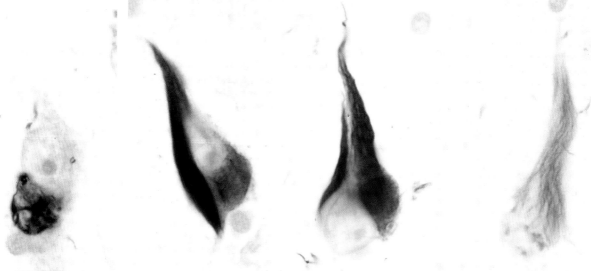

Figure 19 Intraneuronal changes are slow to develop. NFTs change markedly in appearance as they grow to maturity and eventually disappear from the tissue. The first traces of the argyrophilic material are generally seen in close association with intraneuronal lipofuscin deposits (left). Fibrillary masses then fill large portions of the cell body. In some types of neurons, the resulting tangle may extend into the proximal dendrites, but never into the proximal axon. Tangle-bearing neurons eventually die. After deterioration of the parent cell, the pathological material is transformed into a less densely twisted and less argyrophilic extraneuronal 'ghost' or 'tombstone' tangle (right)

changes. Susceptible cells include the glutamatergic, GABAergic, dopaminergic, noradrenergic, adrenergic, serotonergic and cholinergic neurons. In the cerebral cortex, NFT-bearing nerve cells are all included in the class of pyramidal (projection) neurons. Cells furnishing long ipsilateral cortico-cortical connections are particularly prone to

develop NFTs and NTs. The pyramidal cells are sturdy constituents of the cortex and may survive for a long time despite marked cytoskeletal alterations. However, tangle-bearing neurons eventually die for reasons that remain obscure. Following deterioration of the parent cell, the NFT becomes a less densely twisted extraneuronal 'ghost' or

Figure 20 Stage I cortical intra-neuronal change is defined by the appearance of NFTs and NTs in the transentorhinal region. The particularly susceptible cells in this region are closely related to the multiform projection cells in the superficial entorhinal cellular layer

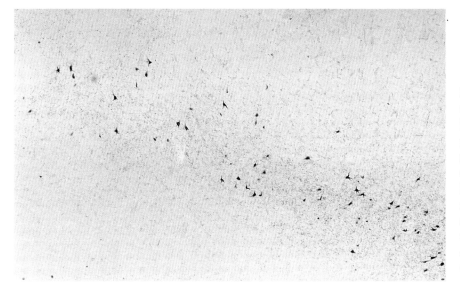

Figure 21 In stage II, the transentorhinal region shows a large number of tangle-bearing projection neurons; there is a gradual involvement of the entorhinal region and Ammon's horn. In stages I and II, the neurofibrillary changes are virtually confined to the guiding components of the limbic system located in the medial portions of the temporal lobe

'tombstone' tangle. The occurrence of such ghost tangles alone has yet to be observed. Fresh NFTs typically accompany the ghost tangles, an indication that, once it has begun, the destructive process progresses relentlessly and immutably. Spontaneous remission does not occur in AD.

Initially, NFTs and NTs develop selectively at specific cortical predilection sites, usually the transentorhinal region. Then, according to a predictable pattern, the destruction extends into the hippocampus and gradually into the neocortex[3]. In general, the poorly myelinated cortical areas develop the changes earlier and to a higher density than the richly myelinated fields[10]. This sequence of changes varies little and thus provides a basis for distinguishing stages in the evolution of the changes.

Interestingly, a number of brains from prospective clinicopathological studies demonstrate a correlation between the results of the neuropathological staging procedure and assessments of the intellectual status of the patient[11–13]. Early stages are seen predominantly in relatively young individuals and the more advanced stages appear with increasing age[14]. However, the initial lesions may develop in a young and otherwise healthy brain; an advanced

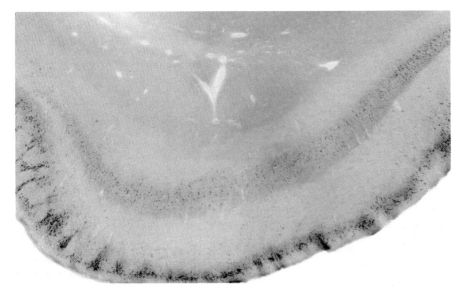

Figure 22 Further progression of AD leads to stage III, with severe involvement of the entorhinal territory, amygdala and hippocampal formation. There is marked destruction of the superficial cellular layer in the entorhinal and transentorhinal regions, and slightly less severe involvement in one of the deep entorhinal layers. Both layers are important as relay stations for the transfer of data from the neocortex to the hippocampal formation and *vice versa*

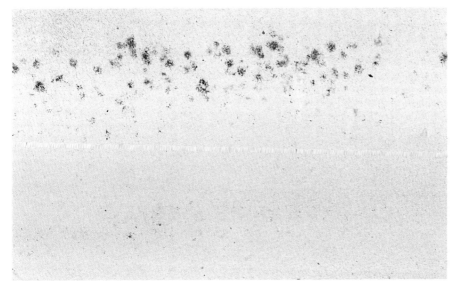

Figure 23 Some cortical areas (for example, the primary sensory fields of the neocortex) are particularly prone to the development of neuritic plaques in the supragranular layers. In these areas, the initial stage IV lesions consist of supragranular neuritic plaques (shown here in the striate area)

age is not a prerequisite for the development of these changes[6].

In AD, stage I is defined as the appearance of the first NFTs and NTs in the transentorhinal region. In stage II, there is already a large number of tangle-bearing neurons at this location, and additional tangles are seen in the entorhinal region and Ammon's horn. Stages I and II are not associated with any obvious impairment of intellectual capacity. As with many other neurodegenerative diseases, the pathological process may be present over an extended period of time before the onset of clinical symptoms. The destruction of the brain slowly progresses until the damage can no longer be compensated for by the individual's reserve capacities. Stages I and II thus represent the clinically silent period of AD (Figures 20 and 21).

Further progression of the disease leads to stages III and IV (Figures 22 and 23) with severe involvement of the entorhinal territory, amygdala and hippocampal formation. At these stages, the transfer of data through the limbic loop is considerably impaired. Particularly ominous is the destruction of the specific external and internal entorhinal layers responsible for data transfer from the neo-cortex to the hippocampal formation and *vice versa*. The local

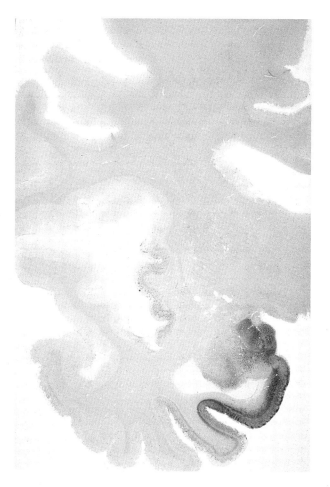

pathological process eventually interrupts the limbic loop at multiple sites (Figure 24). The clinical presentation of many individuals at stage III or IV includes mild impairment of cognitive functions (incipient AD). In others, the appearance of initial symptoms is still camouflaged by a reserve capacity which compensates for the local destruction.

The final stages of AD show large numbers of NFTs / NTs in virtually every subdivision of the cerebral cortex. A key feature of stage V (Figure 25) is a devastating destruction of neocortical association areas. In general, the severity of destruction decreases stepwise proceeding away from the association areas *via* the secondary belt fields into the primary areas. As an example, the boundary

Figure 24 In stage IV, the destructive process has expanded markedly from the entorhinal region into the amygdala, hippocampal formation and, in particular, from the transentorhinal region into the adjoining association areas of the temporal neocortex. Due to the specific bilateral destruction of important limbic areas, many patients with stage III or IV destruction present with the initial clinical symptoms of AD

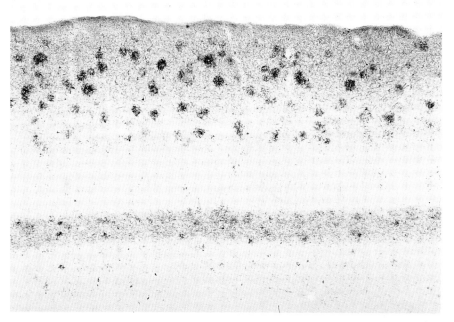

Figure 25 In stage V, a key feature is devastating destruction of the neocortical association areas. A dense network of NTs and numerous inconspicuous NFTs supplement the supragranular neuritic plaques in the striate area. In this case, a dense network of NTs indicates the position of layer V

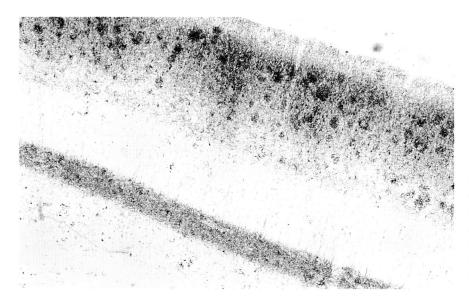

Figure 26 In stage VI, a very high density of NTs is seen in the supragranular layers of the striate area. Layer V is sharply demarcated. In the section here, radially oriented NTs pierce the dense plexus of myelinated fibers (line of Gennari)

between the parastriate field and peristriate region (areas 18 and 19 of Brodmann, respectively), which is not easily detected in the normal human brain, often appears with remarkable clarity in the end-stage of AD.

At stage VI (Figures 26 and 27), even the sensory core fields are severely involved and only the primary motor area continues to exhibit a comparatively low intensity of neurofibrillary changes (Figures 28 and 29). The clinical presentation of stage V or VI in patients generally includes the presence of severe dementia.

Acknowledgements

The authors are grateful for the skillful assistance of Ms Szász with the artwork and of Ms Trautmann for the photography. We also would like to thank the Deutsche Forchungsgemeinschaft (DFG), the Bundesministerium für Bildung, Wissenschaft, Forschung und Tecknologie (BMBF), the Alzheimer Research Center Frankfurt (AFZF), and Degussa / Hanau for their support.

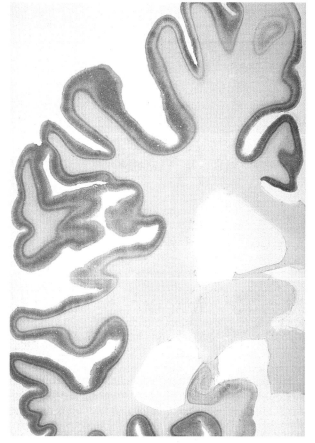

Figure 27 Final stages of AD (stages V and VI) show high densities of neurofibrillary changes in virtually every subdivision of the cerebral cortex. End-stage VI (shown here) is characterized by severe involvement of the entire neocortex

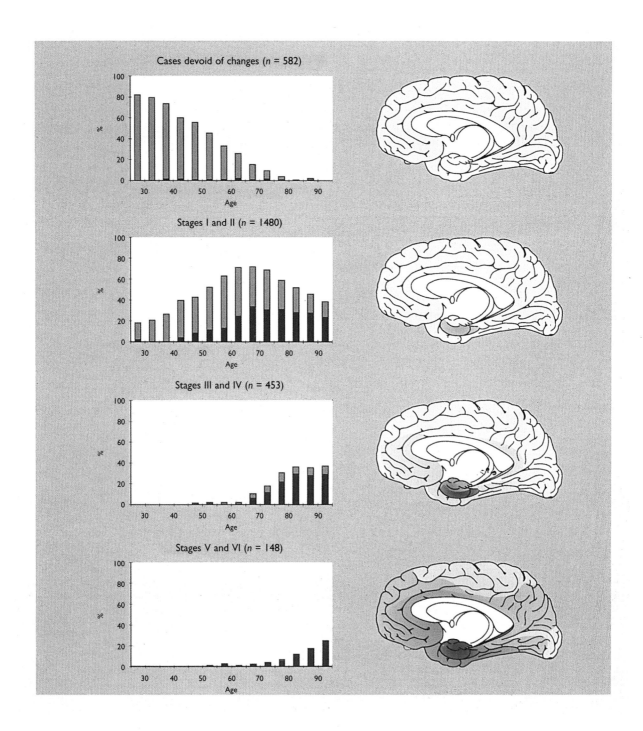

Figure 28 Pattern of distribution of neurofibrillary changes in the course of AD (left). Stages I and II show alterations virtually confined to a single layer of the transentorhinal and entorhinal regions whereas stages III and IV show severe changes in the entorhinal territory and additional involvement of many related limbic structures. Stages V and VI are characterized by devastating destruction of the neocortex. The increasing color intensity reflects the growing density of NFTs and NTs. The graphs show the frequency of stages of AD-related neurofibrillary changes in 2661 non-selected autopsy cases according to age (right), with one subgroup devoid of amyloid deposits (light blue) and another expressing amyloid protein regardless of stage (A–C; dark blue). Reproduced from reference 6, with permission

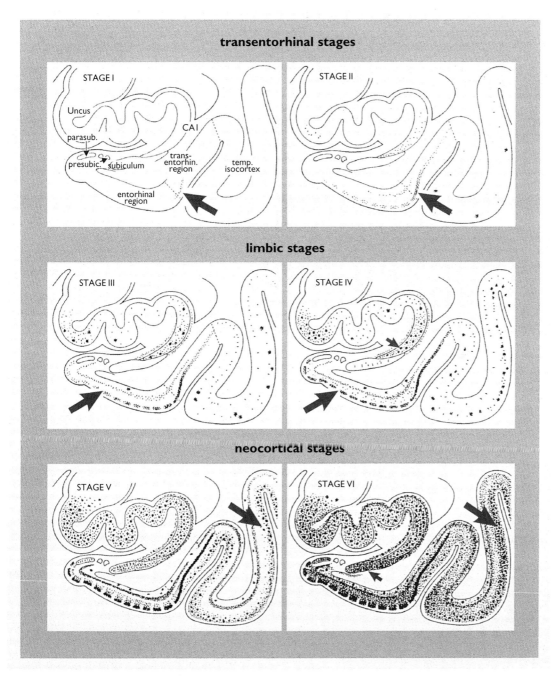

Figure 29 Neurofibrillary changes seen at the level of the uncus in the hippocampal formation, entorhinal and transentorhinal regions, and adjoining temporal neocortex. Note the development of changes from stage I to VI (arrows indicate key features). The changes start in the transentorhinal region (stage I) and extend into the superficial cellular layer of the entorhinal region (stage II). Limbic stages III and IV predominantly involve the entorhinal territory. Destruction of neocortical association areas is the key feature of stage V. The severity of the lesions decreases from the association areas *via* the belt areas to the core fields of the neocortex. At stage VI, even the sensory core fields are severely involved. In addition, many granule cells of the fascia dentata develop tangles and the subiculum displays a remarkably high density of NTs. CA1, first sector of Ammon's horn; entorhin, entorhinal; parasub, parasubiculum; presubic, presubiculum; temp, temporal; transentorhin, transentorhinal. Reproduced from reference 3, with permission

References

1. Braak H, Braak E, Yilmazer D, et al. Pattern of brain destruction in Parkinson's and Alzheimer's diseases. J Neural Transm 1996;103:455–90

2. Braak H, Braak E, Yilmazer D, Bohl J. Functional anatomy of human hippocampal formation and related structures. J Child Neurol 1996;11:265–75

3. Braak H, Braak E. Neuropathological staging of Alzheimer-related changes. Acta Neuropathol 1991; 82:239–59

4. Braak H, Braak E. Pathology of Alzheimer's disease. In: Calne DB, ed. Neurodegenerative Diseases. Philadelphia: WB Saunders, 1994:585–613

5. Duyckaerts C, Delaère P, He Y, et al. The relative merits of tau and amyloid markers in the neuropathology of Alzheimer's disease. In: Bergener M, Finkel SI, eds. Treating Alzheimer's and Other Dementias. New York: Springer-Verlag, 1995:81–9

6. Braak H, Braak E. Frequency of stages of Alzheimer-related lesions in different age categories. Open Peer Commentary. Neurobiol Aging 1997;18:351–7

7. Bancher C, Brunner C, Lassmann H, et al. Accumulation of abnormally phosphorylated τ precedes the formation of neurofibrillary tangles in Alzheimer's disease. Brain Res 1989;477:90–9

8. Braak E, Braak H, Mandelkow EM. A sequence of cytoskeleton changes related to the formation of neurofibrillary tangles and neuropil threads. Acta Neuropathol 1994;87:554–67

9. Braak H, Braak E. Demonstration of amyloid deposits and neurofibrillary changes in whole brain sections. Brain Pathol 1991;1:213–6

10. Braak H, Braak E. Development of Alzheimer-related neurofibrillary changes in the neocortex inversely recapitulates cortical myelogenesis. Acta Neuropathol 1996;92:197–201

11. Bancher C, Braak H, Fischer P, Jellinger KA. Neuropathological staging of Alzheimer lesions and intellectual status in Alzheimer's and Parkinson's disease. Neurosci Lett 1993;162:179–82

12. Duyckaerts C, He Y, Seilhean D, et al. Diagnosis and staging of Alzheimer's disease in a prospective study involving aged individuals. Neurobiol Aging 1994; 15(Suppl 1):140–1

13. Jellinger K, Braak H, Braak E, Fischer P. Alzheimer lesions in the entorhinal region and isocortex in Parkinson's and Alzheimer's diseases. Ann NY Acad Sci 1991;640:203–9

14. Ohm TG, Müller H, Braak H, Bohl J. Close-meshed prevalence rates of different stages as a tool to uncover the rate of Alzheimer's disease-related neurofibrillary changes. Neuroscience 1995;64:209–17

6 Neurofibrillary degeneration
Khalid Iqbal and Inge Grundke-Iqbal

Independent of the etiology – whether genetic or non-genetic – Alzheimer's disease (AD) is characterized by a specific type of neuronal degeneration referred to as neurofibrillary degeneration. The neuronal cytoskeleton in AD is progressively disrupted and replaced by bundles of paired helical filaments (PHFs), also known as neurofibrillary tangles (NFTs)[1,2]. In addition to the neuronal perikaryon, the PHFs also accumulate in the neuropil as neuropil threads (NTs)[3] and as dystrophic neurites surrounding wisps or a core of β-amyloid in neuritic plaques (NPs)[4,5].

At present, the exact relationship between neurofibrillary degeneration and β-amyloidosis, the two hallmark lesions of AD, is not understood. The bulk of the available data suggests that these two lesions are formed independently of each other and that neither is likely to cause the formation of the other in AD (Figure 1). The number of neurons undergoing neurofibrillary degeneration increases with the progression of the disease and correlates with the degree of dementia[6–10]; β-amyloidosis alone without neurofibrillary degeneration does not produce the disease clinically (Figures 2–5). Indeed, some elderly individuals without AD may have as much β-amyloid deposition in their brains as do those who are typical cases of AD. This chapter describes the role of neurofibrillary degeneration in AD.

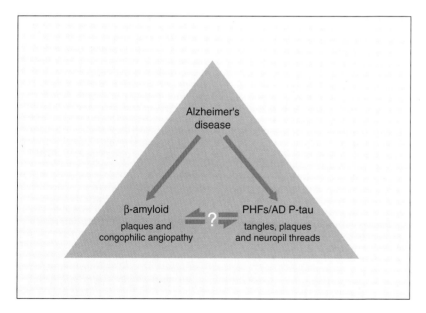

Figure 1 Relationship between neurofibrillary degeneration and β-amyloidosis, the two hallmark lesions of Alzheimer's disease. PHFs, paired helical filaments

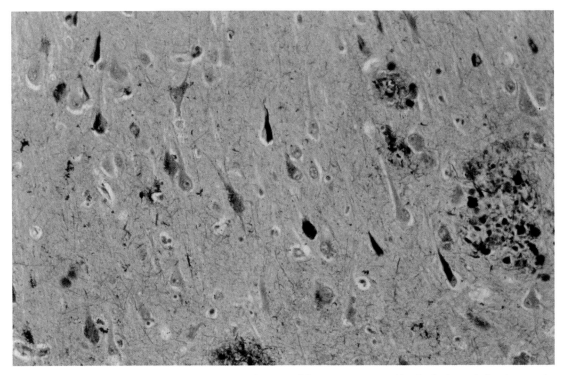

Figure 2 Histological section of hippocampus from an AD patient, stained by Bielschowsky's silver technique, showing neurons with neurofibrillary tangles (NFT), neuropil threads (NT) and neuritic (senile) plaques (NP)

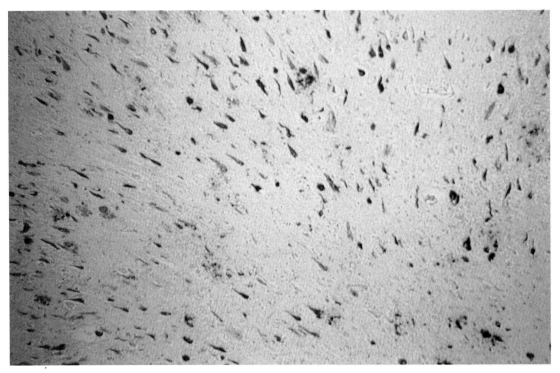

Figure 3 Histological section of hippocampus from an AD patient, immunostained for PHF, shows neurofibrillary tangles (NFT), neuropil threads (NT) and neuritic plaques (NP)

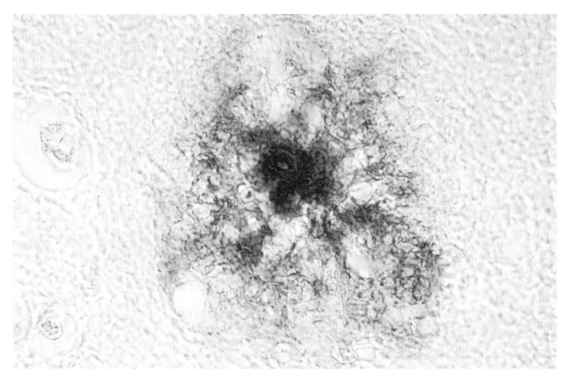

Figure 4 Neuritic (senile) plaque, immunostained with antibody to β-amyloid, shows the amyloid core, but the dystrophic and degenerating neurites at the corona of the plaque remain unstained

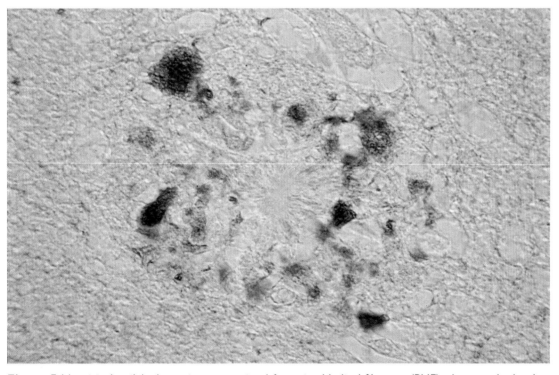

Figure 5 Neuritic (senile) plaque immunostained for paired helical filament (PHF), shows only the dystrophic and degenerating neurites containing accumulations of PHF or its protein subunit, the abnormally hyperphosphorylated tau. β-amyloid, comprising the core of the plaque, is unstained

Topography and morphology

NFTs are intensely stained by silver impregnation techniques and, after staining with Congo red, produce a green birefringence under polarized light (Figure 6). They are found primarily in the cerebral cortex, especially in the hippocampal pyramidal cells of the Sommers sector and in small pyramidal neurons in the outer laminae of the frontotemporal cortex. NFTs have not been seen in the cerebellum, spinal cord and peripheral nervous system. In rare cases, a few NFTs have been reported in astroglial cells.

Unlike the cytoskeleton of a normal mature neuron which is composed mainly of microtubules and neurofilaments (Figures 7–9), NFTs are composed of PHFs (Figures 10–12). A PHF is around

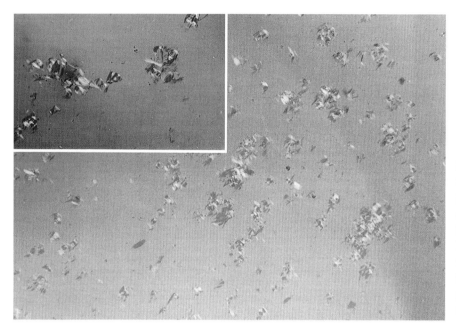

Figure 6 Neurofibrillary tangles isolated from the neocortex of an AD brain by the method described in Iqbal *et al. Acta Neuropathol (Berl)* 1984;62:167–77, stained with Congo red and visualized under partially polarized light. Apple-green birefringence is typical of β-pleated sheet proteins

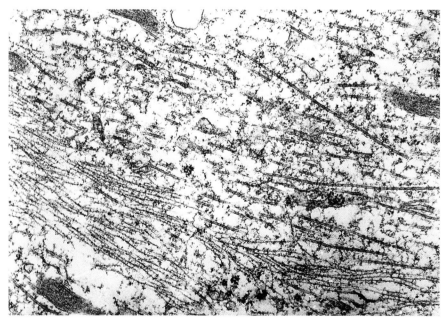

Figure 7 Electron micrograph of normal neuronal cytoskeleton, which is composed of neurofilaments and microtubules in a normal neuronal process. ×95 000. Reproduced from Iqbal K *et al.* Neurofibrillary pathology: An update. In: Nandy K, Sherwin I, eds. *The Aging Brain and Senile Dementia.* New York: Plenum Publishing Co.,1977, with permission

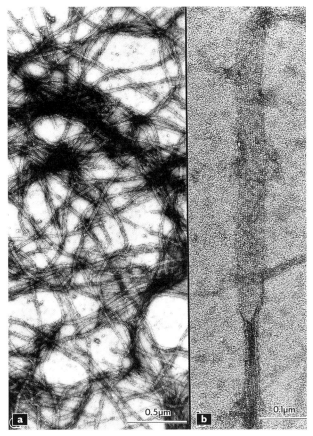

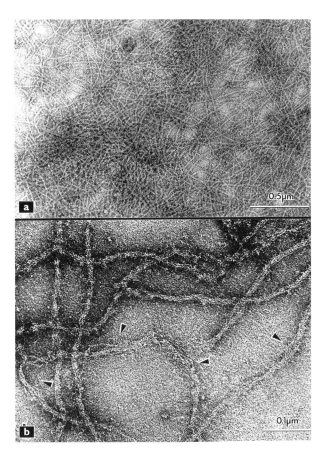

Figure 8 Electron micrograph of assembled microtubules *in vitro* from brain, negatively stained with uranyl acetate, at low (a) and high (b) magnification. The protofilamentous structure of the microtubule is readily apparent in the opened portion (b). Reproduced from Wisniewski, Merz & Iqbal. *J Neuropathol Exp Neurol* 1984;43:643–56, with permission

Figure 9 Electron micrograph of neurofilaments isolated from brain, negatively stained with uranyl acetate, at low (a) and high (b) magnification shows protofilaments of neurofilaments (arrowed). Reproduced from Wisniewski, Merz & Iqbal. *J Neuropathol Exp Neurol* 1984;43:643–56, with permission

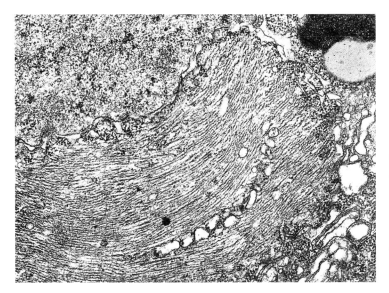

Figure 10 Electron micrograph of a neuron with an NFT from an AD brain shows bundles of PHFs in the neuronal cytoplasm. The neuronal nucleus is on the upper left. × 43 500. Reproduced from Iqbal K *et al.* Neurofibrillary pathology: An update. In: Nandy K, Sherwin I, eds. *The Aging Brain and Senile Dementia.* New York: Plenum Publishing Co.,1977, with permission

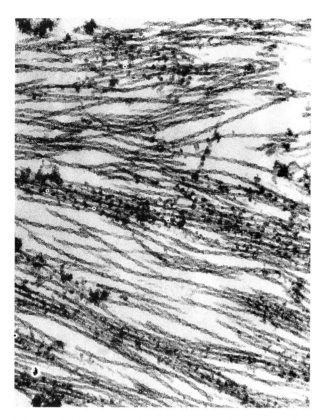

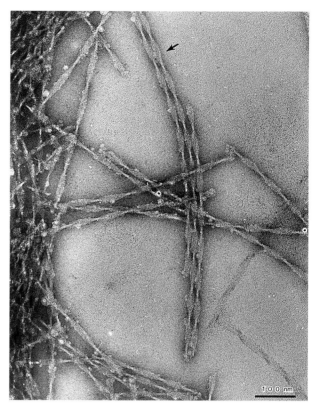

Figure 11 Electron micrograph of an NFT in an AD brain. The PHFs are several microns in length with twists every ~80 mm along its length. × 77 000

Figure 12 Electron micrograph of PHFs isolated from the neocortex of an AD brain by the method described in Iqbal *et al. Acta Neuropathol (Berl)* 1984;62:167–77 and negatively stained with phosphotungstic acid. Four protofilaments are seen along the length of the PHF (arrowed)

20–22 nm in diameter and twisted approximately every 80 nm to an apparent diameter of around 10 nm[11,12]; its structure is heterogeneous. Both the paired-filament and twisted-ribbon forms have been reported to have different narrow and wide regions and periodicities[13]. In neurons undergoing neurofibrillary changes, PHFs appear to become gradually more densely packed and come to occupy a large proportion of the cell space while displacing cytoplasmic organelles. There is little turnover, if any, of these NFTs in neurons. Many of the affected neurons eventually die, leaving the NFTs behind as 'tombstones' or 'ghost tangles' floating in the extracellular space.

Type and distribution of NFTs

Although NFTs composed of PHFs are most com-

monly associated with AD, they are found in small numbers in the entorhinal cortex of non-demented elderly subjects, and in great abundance in the Guam Parkinsonian dementia complex, dementia pugilistica, postencephalitic Parkinsonism and adults with Down syndrome. This lesion has also been observed in small numbers in several cases of subacute sclerosing panencephalitis (SSPE), in rare cases of Hallervorden–Spatz disease and in juvenile neurovisceral lipid storage disease[14]. PHF is rarely formed in animals, with the exception of aged cows[15], sheep[16,17] and goats[17] in which a few of these lesions have been observed. All attempts to form PHF experimentally in animals, including transgenic mice, have thus far proved unsuccessful.

The neurofibrillary changes in human disorders are not always of the AD type (comprising PHF).

In progressive supranuclear palsy, also called Steele–Richardson–Olszewski syndrome, some of the same neurons containing tangles of PHF in an AD brain in fact have tangles composed of 15-nm straight filaments[18] that are sometimes admixed with PHF[19]. In sporadic motor neuron disease, vincristine neuropathy and infantile neuroaxonal dystrophy in humans, the neurofibrillary changes are in the form of neurofilaments. NFTs are also inducible in a few species of animals by aluminum; mitotic spindle inhibitors such as colchicine, vinblastine and podophyllotoxin; various nitrates; and acrylamide (for a review, see reference 20). The aluminum-induced filamentous accumulations are apparently specific to the nervous system whereas, in the case of mitotic spindle inhibitors, similar changes are seen in a wide range of cell types.

Mechanisms of neurofibrillary degeneration and NFT formation

Neurons with NFTs lack microtubules, and microtubule assembly from AD brain cytosol is not observed[21]. PHFs are composed mainly of the microtubule-associated protein (MAP) tau in an abnormally hyperphosphorylated state[22,23]. In addition to PHF, there is a pool of cytosolic abnormally phosphorylated tau protein in the affected neurons[21,24]. This pool of abnormal tau, seen immunocytochemically as 'stage 0' tangles[25], is most likely the precursor of PHF as NFTs have very little turnover, if any, and survive even after the death of the affected neurons.

Tau promotes the assembly of tubulin into microtubules and maintains microtubular structure. Microtubules, in turn, are required for axonal transport. These functions of tau are regulated by its degree of phosphorylation. Normal brain tau, which is optimally active, has 2–3 mol of phosphate per mole of the protein. Tau in PHFs and in an AD brain (AD P-tau), which is abnormally hyperphosphorylated, contains 5–9 mol of phosphate per mole of tau protein[24]. Unlike normal tau, AD P-tau does not promote *in-vitro* assembly of microtubules, bind to microtubules nor stabilize their structure[26–28] (Figures 13 and 14). The AD P-tau competes with tubulin in binding to normal tau and inhibits the

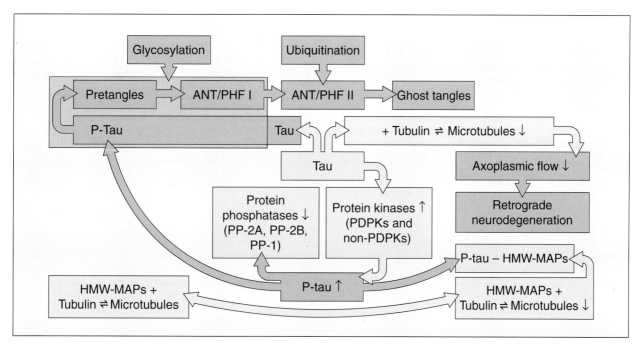

Figure 13 Process by which tau protein becomes hyperphosphorylated in AD and causes neurofibrillary degeneration on sequestration of normal microtubule-associated proteins (MAPs). ANT, Alzheimer neurofibrillary tangle; PHF, paired helical filament; HMW, high molecular weight

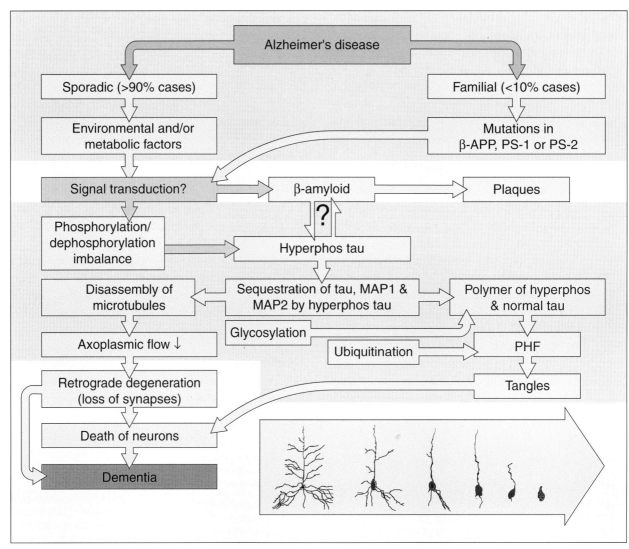

Figure 14 Etiology and pathogenesis of AD. Its polyetiology is characterized by displacement and replacement of the normal cytoskeleton by NFTs of PHFs in the neurons (neurofibrillary degeneration), and deposition of β-amyloid in the extracellular space in the brain parenchyma and in the walls of cerebral vessels (congophilic angiopathy). Neurofibrillary degeneration and β-amyloid are characteristic of, but not unique to, AD. Although both lesions are seen independently of each other, in several other related disorders, neurodegeneration is not inevitably associated with these lesions. In Huntington's chorea, Creutzfeldt–Jakob disease and multi-infarct dementia, neither neurofibrillary degeneration nor β-amyloidosis occur. At present, the nature of the signal transduction pathway that leads to abnormal hyperphosphorylation of tau and β-amyloid is not understood, and there is no compelling evidence that either of the two lesions leads to the other. Unlike normal tau, the abnormally phosphorylated tau does not stimulate assembly of tubulin into microtubules but, instead, inhibits assembly and causes disassembly of microtubules by sequestering normal tau, MAP1 and MAP2. Breakdown of the microtubule network leads to compromised axoplasmic transport and, thus, retrograde degeneration resulting in loss of synapses (affecting neurotransmission and leading to onset of dementia). The association of abnormally hyperphosphorylated tau with normal tau, but not MAP1 or MAP2 in the presence of glycosylation, leads to the formation of NFTs of PHFs. The affected neurons mount what appears to be a largely unsuccessful attempt to degrade the NFTs by ubiquitination. With time, the NFTs come to occupy more and more of the cell cytoplasm which eventually leads to the death of the affected neuron. The NFT is left behind as the 'tombstone' in the extracellular space. Modified from Iqbal K and Grundke-Iqbal I. *Mol Psychiatr* 1997;5:175–6

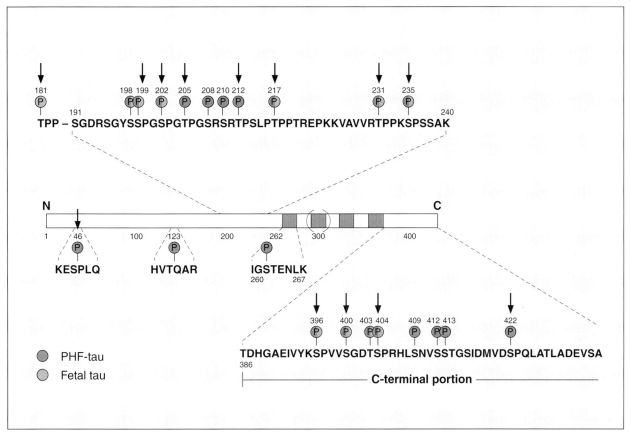

Figure 15 Phosphorylation sites of PHF tau and fetal tau. Ten of the 21 sites in PHF-tau are canonical sites for the proline-directed protein kinases (PDPKs); the remaining 11 sites are non-PDPK sites. Microtubule binding repeats are indicated by the squares. Three of the human tau isoforms have four repeats (T4L, T4S, T4) and the remaining three have three repeats (T3L, T3S, T3)

assembly of microtubules. The association of AD P-tau with normal tau results in tangles of around 3.3 nm straight filaments. Unlike normal tau, AD P-tau is glycosylated, and deglyosylation of AD NFTs by endoglycosidase F / N-glycosidase F converts them into tangles of thin straight filaments[29] similar to those formed by the association of AD P-tau and normal tau[28].

In addition to tau, the neuron contains high-molecular-weight (HMW)-MAPs MAP1 and MAP2, which also promote microtubule assembly and maintain the structure of microtubules. As with tau, MAP1 and MAP2 are associated with AD P-tau, and sequestration of HMW-MAPs from microtubules by AD P-tau results in microtubule disassembly[30]. Both the disassembly of microtubules and the sequestration of tau, MAP1 and MAP2 by

AD P-tau are inhibited by its dephosphorylation. However, the affinity of the binding between AD P-tau and normal tau is greater than that between AD P-tau and HMW-MAPs. Furthermore, unlike the association between AD P-tau and normal tau, the binding of AD P-tau to MAP1 or MAP2 does not result in the formation of tangles or discrete long filaments. This explains the degeneration of many neurites in the absence of accumulation of PHF in the AD brain. HMW-MAPs have not been observed in isolated PHFs.

Regulation of hyperphosphorylation of tau during neurodegeneration

Tau in PHF is phosphorylated in at least 21 sites[31,32] (Figure 15). Ten of the 21 sites are canonical for proline-directed protein kinases (PDPKs) and the remainder are non-PDPK sites. The sites among these 21 at which phosphorylation converts tau to a toxic protein and protein kinases and protein phosphatases that regulate the phosphorylation at these sites remain to be established. Tau may be phosphorylated by several PDPKs and non-PDPKs[33-40]. Phosphorylation of tau by cdk5, followed by GSK-3 at Thr-231 and Ser-262, account for approximately 60% of the inhibition of its binding to microtubules[39]. CaM kinase II is one of the major kinases that phosphorylates tau *in vivo* at Ser-262[41]. However, thus far, the activities of none of these kinases have been demonstrated to be upregulated in AD.

Phosphorylation of a protein is the function of the activities of protein kinases as well as of the protein phosphatases that regulate the phosphorylation. The hyperphosphorylation of AD P-tau may be the result of either higher activities of protein kinases or lower activities of protein phosphatases, or both. A large number of phosphoprotein phosphatases has been described in mammalian tissues[42]. These enzymes may be divided into two broad types: phosphoseryl / phosphothreonyl-protein phosphatases (PSPs) and phosphotyrosyl protein phosphatases (PTPs). PSPs are further subclassified into four subtypes: protein phosphatase (PP)-1; PP-2A; PP-2B; and PP-2C. These phosphatase activities differ in substrate specificity, dependence on divalent cations and sensitivity to specific inhibitors[42,43]. So far, only phosphorylation of serines and threonines has been observed in both normal tau and AD P-tau. Thus, only PSPs are expected to dephosphorylate tau.

Site-specific dephosphorylation of AD P-tau has been investigated, using phosphorylation-dependent antibodies to tau[44-48]. The AD P-tau is rapidly dephosphorylated by PP-2B at the abnormal sites Ser 46, Ser 198 / Ser 199 / Ser 202, Thr 231, Ser 235 and Ser 396 / Ser 404, by PP-2A at all the above sites except Ser 235, and by PP-1 at only Ser 198 / Ser 199 / Ser 202, Thr 231 and Ser 396 / Ser 404. The activities of all three of these phosphatases (PP-2B, PP-2A and PP-1) in relation to abnormally phosphorylated tau are markedly increased by the presence of Mn^{2+}. Unlike tau *in vitro* phosphorylated by

MAP kinase[49], which is the preferred substrate for $PP-2A_1$ compared with $PP-2A_2$, the AD P-tau is an equally good substrate for both isoforms of PP-2A. No dephosphorylation of abnormal tau by PP-2C has been detected at any of the above sites.

Rapid dephosphorylation of AD P-tau by alkaline phosphatase[21,23,50], and by PP-2A, PP-2B and PP-1[44-46] *in vitro* suggested that the abnormal hyperphosphorylation of tau may be, in part, the result of a deficiency of the phosphoprotein phosphatase system in the brains of AD patients. To have a direct effect on the regulation of phosphorylation of tau, PP-2A, PP-2B and PP-1 need to be present in the affected neurons. Immunocytochemical studies have revealed that these PPs are present in both granular and pyramidal neurons, including the tangle-bearing neurons[51]. Using ^{32}P-labeled (with protein kinase A) phosphorylase kinase as substrate and specific inhibitors, it has been shown that the activities of PP-1, PP-2A, PP-2B and PP-2C can be determined in autopsied (2–7 h) and frozen human brains, and that the activities of PP-1 and PP-2A are decreased in an AD neocortex[52]. Furthermore, dephosphorylation studies of abnormally phosphorylated AD P-tau have revealed that PP-2A and PP-2B and, to a lesser extent, PP-1 are all involved in the dephosphorylation of tau. In addition, the phosphatase activity towards dephosphorylation of Ser 198 / Ser 199 / Ser 202, major abnormal phosphorylation sites in the abnormal tau, is decreased by 30% in the brain of patients with AD[53].

In addition to the activities of protein kinases and protein phosphatases, the phosphorylation of tau may also be regulated at the substrate level. In the human brain, there are six molecular isoforms of tau which are all products of a single gene and the result of alternate splicing of its messenger RNA (mRNA). These six tau isoforms differ from one another by having three (τ3L, τ3S, τ3) or four (τ4L, τ4S, τ4) microtubule binding repeats of 31 amino acids each, and by having none (τ3, τ4), one (τ3S, τ4S) or two (τ3L, τ4L) amino terminal inserts of 29 amino acids each[54]. Tau proteins with two amino terminal inserts (τ3L, τ4L) are more favorable substrates than those without these inserts (τ3, τ4) for phosphorylation by cdk5 plus GSK-3, and phosphorylation by this combination of protein kinases inhibit the binding of tau to microtubules by around 80% (Sengupta et al., in preparation). The substrate-dependent regulation of phosphorylation of tau may play a significant role in AD and related neurodegenerative conditions such as in certain genetic cases of frontotemporal / inherited dementias[55–57].

Dephosphorylation by PP-2A, PP-2B and, to a lesser extent, PP-1 restores the microtubule assembly-promoting activity of AD P-tau[48]. Furthermore, the dephosphorylation of NFTs comprising PHF by the two major tau phosphatases, PP-2A and PP-2B, produces marked biochemical, biological and structural alterations[47]. Both PP-2A and PP-2B dephosphorylate PHF-tau at Ser 198 / Ser 199 / Ser 202 and result in only partial dephosphorylation at Ser 396 / Ser 404; in addition, PHF-tau is dephosphorylated at Ser 46 by PP-2A, and at Ser 235 by PP-2B.

The relative electrophoretic mobility of PHF-tau increases after dephosphorylation by either enzyme. Divalent cations, manganese and magnesium increase the activities of PP-2A and PP-2B towards PHF-tau. Dephosphorylation by both PP-2B and PP-2A decreases the resistance of PHF-tau to proteolysis by the brain calcium-activated neutral proteases, the calpains. The capability of PHF-tau to promote microtubule assembly in vitro is restored after dephosphorylation by $PP-2A_1$ and PP-2B. Microtubules assembled by dephosphorylated PHF-tau are structurally identical to those assembled by normal tau. The dephosphorylation both by $PP-2A_1$ and PP-2B causes dissociation of the tangles and the PHF, and some of the PHFs dissociate into straight protofilaments / subfilaments. Approximately 25% of the total tau is released from the PHFs on dephosphorylation by $PP-2A_1$.

These observations have demonstrated that tau in PHFs is accessible to dephosphorylation by $PP-2A_1$ and PP-2B, and dephosphorylation causes PHF to dissociate, and become accessible to proteolysis by calpain and biologically active in promoting the assembly of tubulin into microtubules. Thus, a decrease of tau phosphatase activity could be the cause of the abnormal hyperphosphorylation of tau in AD. By increasing the activities of one or more of these tau phosphatases, it might be possible to prevent and inhibit neuronal degeneration and, consequently, both sporadic as well as familial AD.

Acknowledgements

We thank Ms Janet Biegelson for her secretarial assistance and the Biomedical Photography Unit for their preparation of the Figures

Our studies were supported in part by the New York State Office of Mental Retardation and Developmental Disabilities, and by National Institutes of Health grants AG 05892, AG 08076 and NS 18105.

References

1. Kidd M. Alzheimer's disease: an electron microscopical study. Brain 1964;87:307–20

2. Terry RD, Gonatas NK, Weiss M. Ultrastructural studies in Alzheimer's presenile dementia. Am J Pathol 1964;44:269–97

3. Braak H, Braak E, Grundke-Iqbal I, et al. Occurrence of neuropil threads in the senile human brain and in Alzheimer's disease: A third location of paired helical filaments outside of neurofibrillary tangles and neuritic plaques. Neurosci Lett 1986;65:351–5

4. Wisniewski HM, Terry RD. Morphology of the aging brain, human and animal. Prog Brain Res 1973;40:184–6

5. Glenner GG, Wong CW. Alzheimer's disease and Down's syndrome: sharing of a unique cerebrovascular amyloid fibril protein. Biochem Biophys Res Commun 1984;122:1131–5

6. Tomlinson BE, Blessed G, Roth M. Observations on the brains of demented old people. J Neurol Sci 1970;11:205–42

7. Alafuzoff I, Iqbal K, Friden H, *et al.* Histopathological criteria for progressive dementia disorders: clinical-pathological correlation and classification by multivariate data analysis. *Acta Neuropathol (Berl)* 1987;74:209–25

8. Arrigada PA, Growdon JH, Hedley-White ET, *et al.* Neurofibrillary tangles but not senile plaques parallel duration and severity of Alzheimer's disease. *Neurology* 1992;42:631–9

9. Dickson DW, Crystal HA, Mattiace LA, *et al.* Identification of normal and pathological aging in prospectively studied nondemented elderly humans. *Neurobiol Aging* 1991;13:179–89

10. Barcikowska M, Wisniewski HM, Bancher C, *et al.* About the presence of paired helical filaments in dystrophic neurites participating in the plaque formation. *Acta Neuropathol* 1989;78:225–31

11. Kidd M. Paired helical filaments in electron microscopy of Alzheimer's disease. *Nature* 1963;197:192–3

12. Wisniewski HM, Narang HK, Terry RD. Neurofibrillary tangles of paired helical filaments. *J Neurol Sci* 1976;27:173–81

13. Ruben GC, Iqbal K, Grundke-Iqbal I, *et al.* The organization of the microtubule associated protein tau in Alzheimer paired helical filaments. *Brain Res* 1993;602:1–13

14. Wisniewski K, Jergis GA, Moretz RC, *et al.* Alzheimer neurofibrillary tangles in diseases other than senile and presenile dementia. *Ann Neurol* 1979;5:288–94

15. Nelson PT, Stefansson K, Gulcher J, *et al.* Molecular evolution of tau protein: implications for Alzheimer's disease. *J Neurochem* 1996;67:1622–32

16. Nelson PT, Saper CB. Ultrastructure of neurofibrillary tangles in the cerebral cortex of sheep. *Neurobiol Aging* 1995;16:315–23

17. Braak H, Braak E, Strothjohann M. Abnormally phosphorylated tau proteins related to the formation of neurofibrillary tangles and neuropils threads in cerebral cortex of sheep and goat. *Neurosci Lett* 1994;171:1–4

18. Tellez-Nagle I, Wisniewski HM. Ultrastructure of neurofibrillary tangles in Steele–Richardson–Olszewski syndrome. *Arch Neurol* 1973;29:324–7

19. Ghatak NR, Nochlin D, Hadfield M.G. Neurofibrillary pathology in progressive supranuclear palsy. *Acta Neuropathol* 1980;52:73–6

20. Wisniewski HM, Terry RD. Neurofibrillary pathology. *J Neuropathol Exp Neurol* 1970;39:163–76

21. Iqbal K, Grundke-Iqbal I, Zaidi T, *et al.* Defective brain microtubule assembly in Alzheimer's disease. *Lancet* 1986;2:421–6

22. Grundke-Iqbal I, Iqbal K, Quinlan M, *et al.* Microtubule-associated protein tau: A component of Alzheimer paired helical filaments. *J Biol Chem* 1986;261:6084–9

23. Grundke-Iqbal I, Iqbal K, Tung Y-C, *et al.* Abnormal phosphorylation of the microtubule associated protein (tau) in Alzheimer cytoskeletal pathology. *Proc Natl Acad Sci USA* 1986;83:4913–7

24. Köpke E, Tung Y-C, Sheikh S, *et al.* Microtubule associated protein tau: abnormal phosphorylation of a non-paired helical filament pool in Alzheimer disease. *J Biol Chem* 1993;268:24374–83

25. Bancher C, Brunner C, Lassmann H, *et al.* Accumulation of abnormally phosphorylated tau precedes the formation of neurofibrillary tangles in Alzheimer's disease. *Brain Res* 1989;477:90–9

26. Iqbal K, Zaidi T, Bancher C, *et al.* Alzheimer paired helical filaments: Restoration of the biological activity by dephosphorylation. *FEBS Lett* 1994;349:104–8

27. Alonso A del C, Zaidi T, Grundke-Iqbal I, *et al.* Role of abnormally phosphorylated tau in the breakdown of microtubules in Alzheimer disease. *Proc Natl Acad Sci USA* 1994;91:5562–6

28. Alonso A del C, Grundke-Iqbal I, Iqbal K. Alzheimer's disease hyperphosphorylated tau sequesters normal tau into tangles of filaments and disassembles microtubules. *Nature Med* 1996;2:783–7

29. Wang J-Z, Grundke-Iqbal, Iqbal K. Glycosylation of microtubule-associated protein tau: An abnormal post-translational modification in Alzheimer's disease. *Nature Med* 1996;2:871–5

30. Alonso A del C, Grundke-Iqbal I, Barra HS, *et al.* Abnormal phosphorylation of tau and the mechanism of Alzheimer neurofibrillary degeneration: Sequestration of MAP1 and MAP2 and the disassembly of microtubules by the abnormal tau. *Proc Natl Acad Sci USA* 1997;94:298–303

31. Morishima-Kawashima M, Hasegawa M, Takio K, *et al.* Hyperphosphorylation of tau in PHF. *Neurobiol Aging* 1995;16:365–80

32. Iqbal K, Grundke-Iqbal I. Alzheimer abnormally phosphorylated tau is more hyperphosphorylated than the fetal tau and causes the disruption of microtubules. *Neurobiol Aging* 1995;16:375–9

33. Baudier J, Cole D. Phosphorylation of tau proteins to a state like that in Alzheimer's brain is catalyzed by a calcium/calmodulin-dependent kinase and modulated by phospholipds, *J Biol Chem* 1987; 262: 17577–83

34. Drewes G, Lichtenberg-Kraag B, Döring F, *et al.* Mitogen activated protein (MAP) kinase transforms tau protein into an Alzheimer-like state. *EMBO J* 1992;11:2131–8

35. Ishiguro K, Takamatsu M, Tomizawa K, *et al.* Tau protein kinase I converts normal tau protein into A68-like component of paired helical filaments. *J Biol Chem* 1992;267:10897–901

36. Ledesma MD, Correas I, Avila J, *et al.* Implication of brain cdc2 and MAP2 kinases in the phosphorylation of tau protein in Alzheimer's disease. *FEBS Lett* 1992;308:218–24

37. Litersky JM, Johnson GVW. Phosphorylation by cAMP-dependent protein kinase inhibits the degradation of tau by calpain. *J Biol Chem* 1992;267:1563–8

38. Roder HM, Ingram VM. Two novel kinases phosphorylate tau and KSP site of heavy neurofilament subunits in high stoichiometric ratios. *J Neurosci* 1991;11:3325–43

39. Sengupta A, Kabat J, Novak M, *et al.* Phosphorylation of tau at both Thr 231 and Ser 262 is regulated for maximal inhibition of its binding to microtubules. *Arch Biochem Biophys* 1998;357:299–309

40. Singh TJ, Grundke-Iqbal I, McDonald B, *et al.* Comparison of the phosphorylation of microtubule associated protein tau by non-proline dependent protein kinases. *Mol Cell Biochem* 1994;131:181–9

41. Sironi J, Yen S-H, Gondal JA, *et al.* Ser 262 in human recombinant tau protein is a markedly more favorable site for phosphorylation by CaMKII than PKA or PhK. *FEBS Lett* 1998;436:471–5

42. Cohen P. The structure and regulation of protein phosphatases. *Ann Rev Biochem* 1989;58:453–508

43. Ingebritsen TS, Cohen P. The protein phosphatases involved in cellular regulation. Classification and substrate specificities. *Eur J Biochem* 1983;132:255–61

44. Gong C-X, Singh TJ, Grundke-Iqbal I, *et al.* Alzheimer disease abnormally phosphorylated tau is dephosphorylated by protein phosphatase 2B (calcineurin). *J Neurochem* 1994;62:803–6

45. Gong C-X, Grundke-Iqbal I, Iqbal K. Dephosphorylation of Alzheimer disease abnormally phosphorylated tau by protein phosphatase-2A. *Neuroscience* 1994;61:765–72

46. Gong C-X, Grundke-Iqbal I, Damuni Z, *et al.* Dephosphorylation of microtubule-associated protein tau by protein phosphatase-1 and -2C and its implication in Alzheimer disease. *FEBS Lett* 1994; 341:94–8

47. Wang J-Z, Gong C-X, Zaidi T, *et al.* Dephosphorylation of Alzheimer paired helical filaments by protein phosphatase-2A and -2B. *J Biol Chem* 1995; 270: 4854–60

48. Wang J-Z, Grundke-Iqbal I, Iqbal K. Restoration of biological activity of Alzheimer abnormally phosphorylated t by dephosphorylation with protein phosphatase-2A, -2B and -1. *Mol Brain Res* 1996;38:200–8

49. Goedert M, Cohen ES, Jakes R, *et al.* 42P map kinase phosphorylation sites in microtubule-associated protein tau are dephosphorylated by protein phosphatase 2A1: Implications for Alzheimer's disease. *FEBS Lett* 1992;312:95–9

50. Iqbal K, Grundke-Iqbal I, Smith AJ, *et al.* Identification and localization of a tau peptide to paired helical filaments of Alzheimer disease. *Proc Natl Acad Sci USA* 1989;86:5646–50

51. Pei J-J, Sersen E, Iqbal K, *et al.* Expression of protein phosphatases PP-1, PP-2A, PP-2B and PTP-1B and

protein kinases MAP kinase and P34cdc2 in the hippocampus of patients with Alzheimer disease and normal aged individuals. *Brain Res* 1994;655:70–6

52. Gong C-X, Singh TJ, Grundke-Iqbal I, *et al.* Phospho-protein phosphatase activities in Alzheimer disease. *J Neurochem* 1993;61:921–7

53. Gong C-X, Shaikh S, Wang J-Z, Zaidi T, *et al.* Phos-phatase activity toward abnormally phosphorylated t: decrease in Alzheimer disease brain. *J Neurochem* 1995;65:732–8

54. Goedert M, Spillanti MG, Jakes R, *et al.* Multiple iso-forms of human microtubule-associated protein tau:

Sequences and localization in neurofibrillary tangles of Alzheimer's disease. *Neuron* 1989;3:519–26

55. Poorkaj P, Bird TD, Wijsman E, *et al.* Tau is a can-didate gene for chromosome 17 frontotemporal dementia. *Ann Neurol* 1994;43:815–25 (1998)

56. Hutton M, Lendon CL, Rizzu P, *et al.* Association of missense and 5'-splice-site mutations in tau with the inherited dementia FTDP-17. *Nature* 1998;393: 702–5

57. Spillantini MG, Murrell JR, Goedert M, *et al.* Mutation in the tau gene in familial multiple system tauopathy with presenile dementia. *Proc Natl Acad Sci USA* 1998; 95:7737–41

7 β-Amyloidosis in Alzheimer's disease

Jerzy Wegiel and Henryk M. Wisniewski

Extracellular β-amyloid (Aβ) deposition in the brain and neurofibrillary degeneration are diagnostic markers of Alzheimer's disease (AD). Aβ is the product of the processing of β-amyloid precursor protein (βPP) encoded by a gene on chromosome 21[1]. Cleavage of βPP with β- and γ-secretases generates β-peptide, which aggregates *in vivo* to produce insoluble β-pleated sheet structures within extracellular amyloid deposits. The synthetic Aβ 1–28, 1–40 or 1–42 peptides form fibrils *in vitro* which morphologically resemble fibrils of natural amyloid detected *in vivo*[2]. Several proteins that are detectable in amyloid deposits – α₁-antichymotrypsin (ACT) [3,4], nucleoside diphosphatase (NDPase)[5], heparan sulfate proteoglycan (HSPG)[6,7], amyloid P component[8,9] and apolipoprotein E (apo E)[10,11] – affect aggregation and fibrilization of Aβ.

AD is found in a sporadic form, with no detectable genetic link, with the onset of dementia after age 60 years and a duration of AD of around 20 years. In its familial form (about 5% of all AD cases), genetic factors influence the age on onset of the disease, the topographical pattern and amount of amyloid deposition, and the duration of AD.

Four genes are now linked to AD. The disease is induced by nine mutations of the βPP gene on chromosome 21, 43 mutations of the presenilin 1 (PS1) gene on chromosome 14 and two mutations of the PS2 gene on chromosome 1. Increased genetic risk for late-onset AD is associated with the gene located on chromosome 19 encoding apo E.

Overexpression of the gene for βPP causes accumulation of a biochemically detectable amount of Aβ42 in the brain of individuals with Down syndrome starting from 21 weeks of gestation[12], followed by the appearance of numerous (60–90/mm²) diffuse Aβ deposits in the neocortex of some Down syndrome patients at around age 15 years, onset of β-amyloidosis with neuritic plaques and amyloid angiopathy, and neurofibrillary degeneration in the brain of all patients with Down syndrome more than 40 years of age[13]. Mutations on chromosome 14 encoding PS1 are associated with extremely early onset of neuritic plaques and amyloid angiopathy (third decade of life), more severe amyloidosis than usually seen in Down syndrome or sporadic AD, and an accelerated course of AD leading to death within approximately 6 years[14,15]. The apo E4/4 allelic form increases both the risk for late onset of AD and amyloid load[16].

The link between the amyloid precursor protein (APP) gene and β-amyloidosis is also shown in several transgenic mouse lines that overexpress variants of the human βPP gene and develop fibrillar thioflavine S-positive Aβ deposits with activated microglia, dystrophic neurites, astrocytosis[17–20] and neuronal loss[21].

Aβ peptides are detectable not only in the brain, but also in blood serum, cerebrospinal fluid (CSF)[22], cultured cells[23] and in the media of cultured cells[23,24]. Messenger RNA (mRNA) for βPP is present in almost all types of cells; however, cellular expression of the gene varies widely. Several types of cells are the source of the extracellular Aβ present in the brain of patients with AD.

Origin of extracellular β-amyloid deposits in Alzheimer's disease

Aβ in the brain is of heterogeneous origin. Morphological classification of amyloid deposition into diffuse Aβ deposits, neuritic plaques, amyloid angiopathy of the capillaries, and amyloid angiopathy of the arteries and veins corresponds to the four sources of Aβ[25]. Some neuronal populations release Aβ which forms diffuse plaques. Perivascular cells of monocyte–macrophage–microglial cell lineage produce fibrillar Aβ in the walls of capillaries whereas parenchymal microglial cells produce fibrillar Aβ in the parenchyma of gray matter. Smooth muscle cells are the source of Aβ in the tunica media of parenchymal and leptomeningeal arteries and veins.

The source of Aβ peptide(s) determines the topography and morphology of deposition, and the type and amount of Aβ and amyloid-associated proteins. These factors in turn determine the cascade of secondary events, including the response of neurons exposed to amyloid and amyloid-associated proteins, activation of glial cells associated with the release of cell-specific cytokines and cytotoxins, and vascular pathology and response to vascular net-

work degradation. A global index of the impact of Aβ pathology on the brain in sporadic AD could be the presence of around 40 plaques / mm² in gray matter or 0.5–1.5 billion plaques in the neocortex. In each neuritic plaque 50–200 μm in diameter, there are several cells engaged in Aβ deposition, and dozens which respond to Aβ deposition by activation and / or degeneration.

Amyloid in diffuse plaque

Diffuse plaque formation is associated with the release of Aβ peptide by neurons[26–30]. In a few brain regions, such as the parvocellular layer of the presubiculum or the molecular layer of the cerebellar cortex, diffuse Aβ deposits are present up to the end-stage of AD.

Presubicular diffuse deposits of Aβ (Figure 1) are thioflavine S- and Congo red-negative; non-fibrillar; and apo E-, apo I-, apo J-, HSPG- and ACT-negative. The absence of activated microglial cells and astrocytes indicates that local glial cells do not react to a heavy (almost 90%) amyloid load. The lack of fibrillar amyloid in diffuse deposits in the presubiculum may be associated with a low concentration of Aβ peptides and / or the absence of chaperon proteins promoting Aβ fibrilization. The presence of neurofibrillary changes in only 2.5% of neurons of the parvopyramidal layer of the presubiculum indicates that Aβ deposition and tau

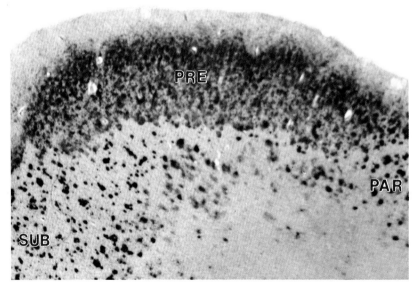

Figure 1 Diffuse non-fibrillar amyloid deposit occupies almost all of the parvopyramidal layer of the presubiculum (PRE) whereas, in the subiculum (SUB) and parasubiculum (PAR), neuritic fibrillar plaques predominate (immunolabeled with mAb 4G8)

pathology coexist in this subregion of the hippocampal formation in a rather benign form. The distinct borders of the presubicular deposits suggest

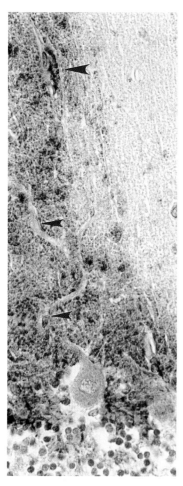

Figure 2 Diffuse Aβ deposits in the dendritic tree (arrowed) of Purkinje cells in the molecular layer of the cerebellar cortex (immunolabeled with mAb 4G8)

that Aβ is the product of projections of one or more neuronal populations to this cytoarchitectonic area.

Diffuse non-fibrillar Aβ deposits without microglial and astrocytic activation and without a neurofibrillar component are present in the molecular layer of the cerebellum for almost 20 years of the duration of AD. A major component of cerebellar plaques is non-amyloidogenic Aβ 17-42 (p3 fragment)[31]. Their topography and distribution suggest that amyloid deposit formation is associated with the dendritic tree of the Purkinje cells (Figure 2).

Non-fibrillar diffuse Aβ deposits are detectable in the outer two-thirds of the molecular layer of the dentate gyrus of subjects with Down syndrome aged 15–40 years. The unique unidirectional innervation of this part of the molecular layer indicates that diffuse Aβ deposits appear in the projection area of one neuronal population, namely, stellate cells in the second layer of the entorhinal cortex. The presence of activated microglial cells, and the formation of fibrillar plaques with neuronal degeneration and astrocytic activation in the molecular layer of the dentate gyrus in persons with Down syndrome aged >40 years and with sporadic AD, indicate that factors of neuronal origin, associated with diffuse Aβ deposition, activate microglial cells and initiate neuritic plaque formation (Figure 3).

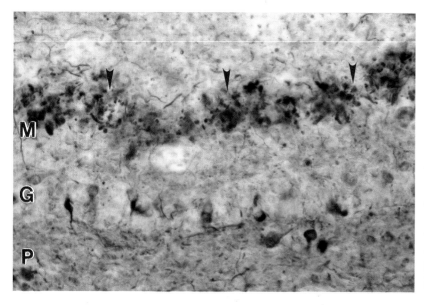

Figure 3 Row of neuritic, fibrillar, tau-positive plaques (arrowed) in the molecular layer (M) of the dentate gyrus. The specific pattern of distribution of plaques suggests that their formation is associated with projections of the stellate cells of the entorhinal cortex to the outer two-thirds of the molecular layer of the dentate gyrus. G, granular layer; P, polymorphic layer (immunolabeled with mAb tau-1)

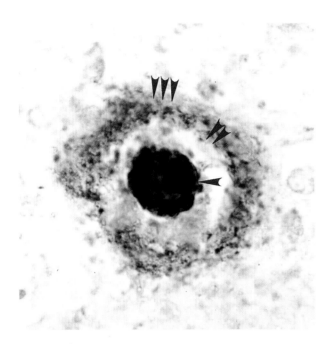

Amyloid in neuritic plaque

Neuritic plaques consist of microglial cells, amyloid, dystrophic neuronal processes and synapses, and astrocytes[32]. In a classical plaque, a centrally positioned amyloid 'star' is surrounded by several microglial cells, dozens of degenerated neurites and synapses, and astrocytic processes (Figures 4 and 5). Primitive plaques consist of one or several microglial cells producing numerous small aggregates of fibrillar Aβ (Figures 6 and 7)[5,33,34].

Figure 4 The classical plaque has an amyloid core in the center (single arrow), a halo (two arrows) and an amyloid corona (three arrows; immunolabeled with mAb 4G8)

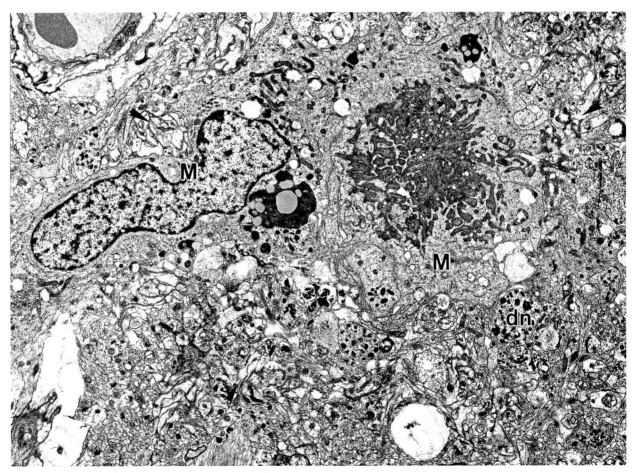

Figure 5 Electron micrograph of the classical plaque with amyloid core surrounded by microglial cells (M). Astrocytic processes are arrowed. dn, dystrophic neurites

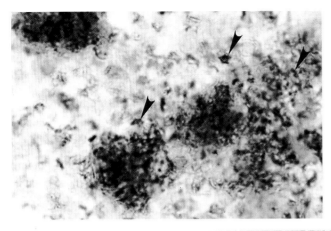

Figure 6 Primitive plaques consist of numerous clusters of Aβ (arrowed; immunolabeled with Mab 4G8)

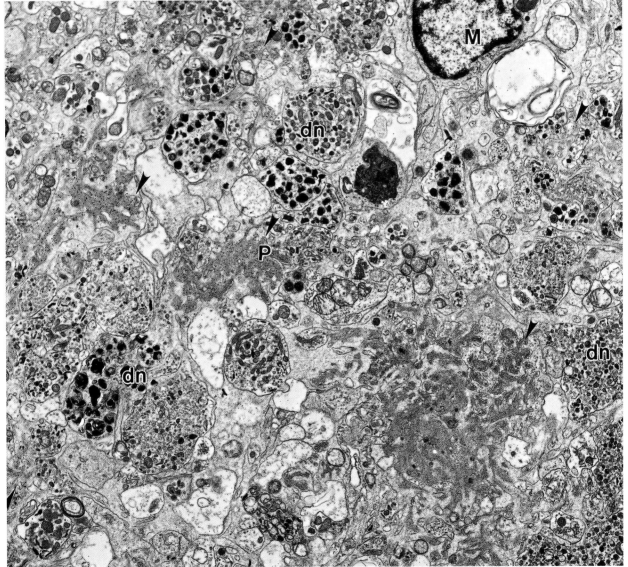

Figure 7 Electron micrograph of a primitive plaque showing a microglial cell (M), clusters of fibrillar amyloid (arrowed) and dystrophic neurites (dn)

Microglial cells in plaques are polarized. The pole facing amyloid deposits bears extensive cell membrane infoldings, which appear to be connected to endoplasmic reticulum (Figure 8)[5,35]. In some cases where cytoplasmic channels are filled with fibrillar Aβ, tubuloreticular structures are detectable. These inclusions are formed in the endoplasmic reticulum of microglial cells, pericytes and endothelial cells. The co-localization of fibrillar amyloid and tubuloreticular structures in the same cytoplasmic channel indicates that amyloid is formed in pathologically altered endoplasmic reticulum[35]. An elaborate system of intracytoplasmic

channels of microglial cells filled with Aβ has numerous connections with extracellular space. Bundles of fibrillar amyloid are secreted from cytoplasmic channels. The presence of bundles of fibrillar amyloid in the cytoplasmic channels, and in unmodified form in the amyloid star periphery and center, suggests that microglial cells form fibrillar amyloid that is stable and relatively resistant to enzymatic degradation. Microglial cells appear to produce highly concentrated Aβ peptides as well as factor(s) promoting Aβ fibrilization and fibril stabilization, such as apo E[36].

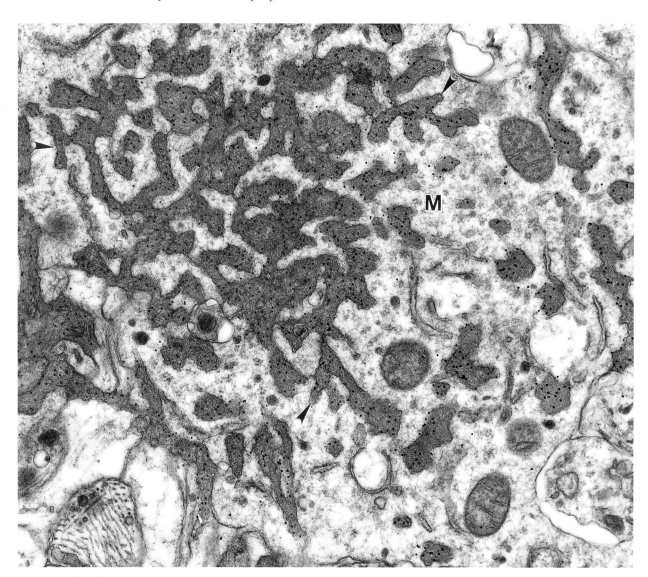

Figure 8 Fibrillar amyloid formation in the deep cytoplasmic channels (arrowed) of a microglial cell (M; immuno-labeled with mAb 4G8)

Amyloid in capillary wall

Experimental studies indicate that parenchymal microglial cells are replaced continuously by blood-borne cells[37], and that perivascular cells enclosed in the vascular basement membrane represent a transitional form between blood monocytes and parenchymal microglial cells[38–40]. In patients with AD, amyloid deposits form hemistars in the capillary walls (Figure 9).

Ultrastructural studies show that perivascular cells and perivascular microglial cells produce fibrillar amyloid in the capillary wall[41,42]. Perivascular cells show the same polarity as parenchymal microglial cells in plaques and have numerous cytoplasmic channels filled with fibrillar Aβ (Figure 10). The effect of the secretory activity of perivascular cells / perivascular microglial cells is local semicircular thickening of the vascular basement membrane, with accumulation of fibrillar Aβ embedded

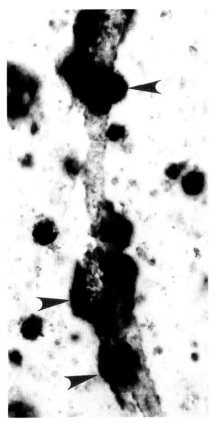

Figure 9 Capillary wall with numerous amyloid hemistars (arrowed)

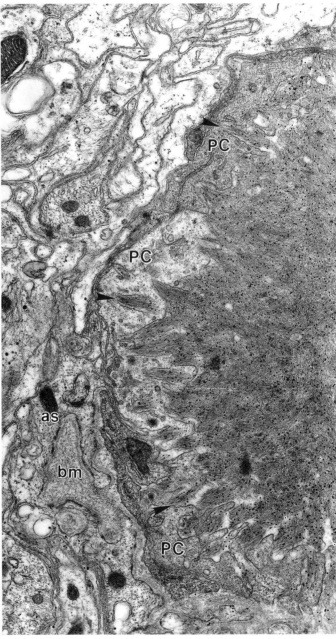

Figure 10 Electron micrograph of the periphery of a hemistar in a capillary wall with fibrillar amyloid formation in the cytoplasmic channels (arrowed) of a perivascular cell (PC). bm, capillary basement membrane; as, astrocytic end foot processes (immunolabeled with mAb 4G8)

in amorphous material of the basement membrane. The morphology of the lesion suggests that perivascular cells produce both proteinaceous material of the basement membrane and fibrillar Aβ. Further production of Aβ causes formation of tuber-like hemistars in the capillary wall. In the hemistar center and periphery, the amount of amorphous material decreases whereas the amount of fibrillar βA increases. During vascular Aβ deposit formation, perivascular cells move into the neuropil and finally lose contact with the vascular wall to become parenchymal microglial cells. Deposition of amyloid by several perivascular cells in close proximity produces a thick amyloid cast in the vascular wall.

Despite some topographic specificity, amyloid deposition by perivascular cells / perivascular microglial cells and parenchymal microglial cells shows striking similarities, indicating that both types of changes are part of the same pathological process.

Amyloid in artery and vein walls

In AD, amyloid accumulates not only in the walls of capillaries, but also in the walls of arteries and – less often – veins. Aβ accumulates in the basement membrane between smooth muscle cells of the tunica media of leptomeningeal and cortical arteries and veins (Figure 11)[43]. Fibrillar amyloid forms thick septa or rings around myocytes (Figure 12).

The first Aβ-positive deposits appear close to the smooth muscle cell membrane in front of rows of sarcolemmal vesicles and, sporadically, in the sarcolemmal vesicles as amorphous material or poorly defined rods or fuzzy fibrils. In the area of amyloid fibrilization, the basal lamina of the muscle cell disappears. As amyloidosis progresses, the number of mature thick fibrils embedded in the abnormally thick, sometimes multilayered, basement membrane increases.

β-Amyloid-associated degeneration

Neuritic plaque

In classical and primitive plaques, the infiltration of neuropil by amyloid fibrils is associated with dystrophic changes in neuronal synapses and dendrites. In neurons with neurofibrillary changes, degeneration is associated with accumulation of paired helical filaments (PHF) in distended synapses and processes in the plaque perimeter (Figure 13, inset). In neurons free of neurofibrillary changes, dystrophic neurites are filled with degenerated

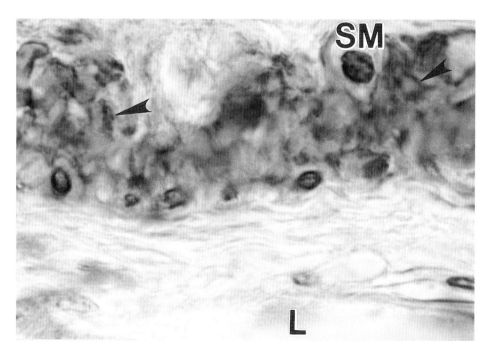

Figure 11 Leptomeningeal artery with amyloid (arrowed) formation between smooth muscle cells (SM) of the tunica media. L, vessel lumen

mitochondria, osmophilic bodies and neurotubules (Figure 13).

The localized nature of the changes with swelling of a short segment of neuronal processes in the plaque perimeter indicates that the pathology is a response to extracellular fibrillar Aβ / amyloid and is associated with changes in the cell membrane. The accumulation of degenerating mitochondria,

osmophilic bodies, neurotubules and PHFs in segments of neuronal processes exposed to amyloid suggests that Aβ affects not only cell membrane, but also cytoplasmic organelles, cell cytoskeleton and transport within neuronal processes. Ultrastructural studies of the neuronal processes and synapses in the plaque perimeter indicate that Aβ is a direct cause of severe impairment of the function of neurons and synapses. The presence of

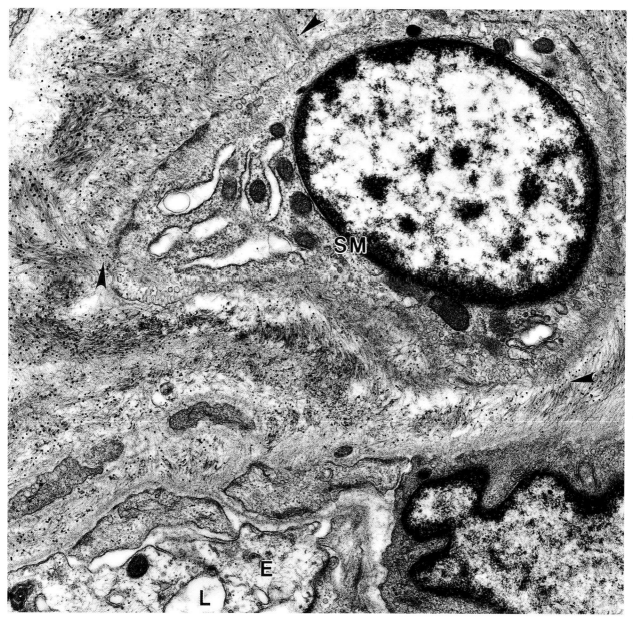

Figure 12 Electron micrograph of the wall of an artery showing a smooth muscle cell (SM) surrounded by a mantle of thick basement membrane with fibrillar amyloid (arrowed). E, endothelial cell; L, vessel lumen (immunolabeled with mAb 4G8)

numerous abnormal synapses and neuronal processes in the plaque perimeter indicates that each plaque is associated with morphological changes and functional impairment of dozens of neurons.

Lack of correlation between the number of plaques and the stage of disease, and the presence of early, mature and old partially degraded plaques in all stages of the disease indicate turnover of neuritic plaques. As a result of formation of new plaques and deterioration of old plaques, with slow degradation of fibrillar amyloid and dead neurons, the local numerical density of plaques may remain unchanged for years. The chronic course of the disease, and the relatively stable number of plaques and their turnover suggest that the damaging effect of plaques may be several times greater than estimated on the basis of the current number of plaques.

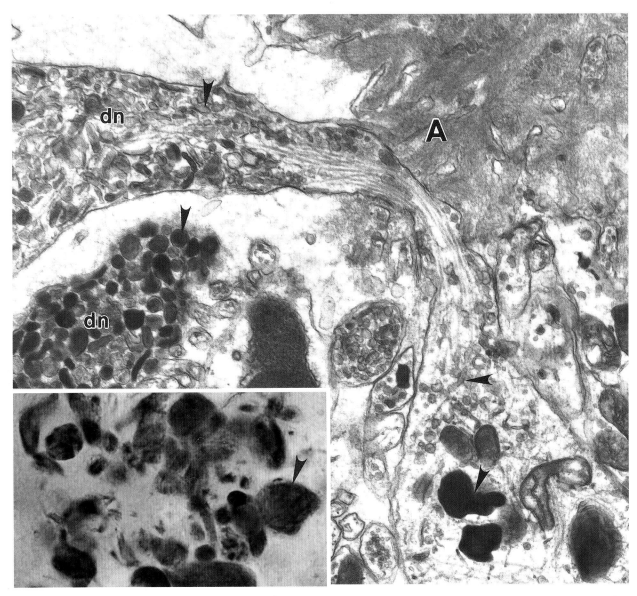

Figure 13 Electron micrograph shows the local response of a neuronal process exposed to direct contact with amyloid (A). Dystrophic neurites (dn) are swollen, and filled with osmophilic bodies and vesicles (arrowed). Segments of neuronal processes in the plaque perimeter (inset) are distended and filled with abnormally phosphorylated tau (arrowed; immunolabeled with mAb tau-1)

β-Amyloid in capillary wall

The direct effects of Aβ deposition by perivascular cells are changes in the wall of capillary vessels with thickening of the capillary basement membrane. Degeneration and death of endothelial cells in the capillary wall infiltrated by Aβ appear to be evidence of the susceptibility of endothelial cells to toxic amyloid deposit components. The lack of neuronal degeneration in the interface between amyloid deposits in the capillary wall and neuropil in the majority of affected vessels suggests that astrocytic end foot processes successfully isolate toxic deposits from neuropil. Proliferation of astrocytic processes around amyloid deposits in the capillary wall indicates that they recognize Aβ and respond with activation without degeneration. Common pathology in the area of capillary amyloidosis includes perivascular edema and hemorrhages.

The lumen of capillary segments affected by amyloidosis is reduced or closed (Figure 14). The secondary effect of obliteration of numerous branches of the capillary tree is local ischemia, with neuronal degeneration and activation of the astrocytes that surround the bodies of degenerating and dying neurons, and degrade cell residues (Figure 15).

β-Amyloid in tunica media of arteries and veins

Fibrillar Aβ deposition in the tunica media of leptomeningeal and parenchymal vessels causes degeneration and necrosis of smooth muscle cells[43]. Aβ deposition starts in the external layer of smooth muscle cells and progresses towards the middle and internal layers. Degenerative changes and loss of smooth muscle cells are usually more severe in the outer zone of the tunica media. Cell debris is removed without detectable involvement of macrophages. Degradation of fibrillar amyloid in the area of smooth muscle cell necrosis indicates that local proteolytic enzymes are present in a sufficiently high concentration as to remove cell residues and Aβ (Figure 16). Degeneration, death and removal of smooth muscle cells contribute to changes in the

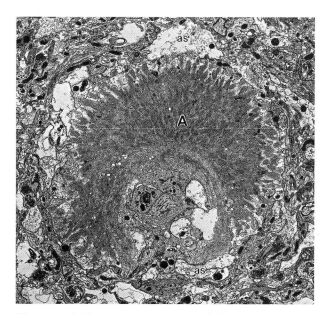

Figure 14 Electron micrograph of the residue of an obliterated capillary including an amyloid hemistar (A) isolated from the neuropil by astrocytic processes (as). No dystrophic neurites are present in the affected area

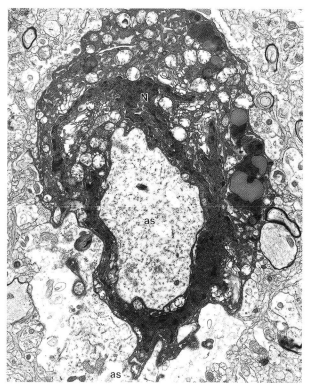

Figure 15 Electron micrograph of an area affected by amyloid angiopathy showing the body of a dying neuron (N) intertwined with swollen astrocytic processes (as)

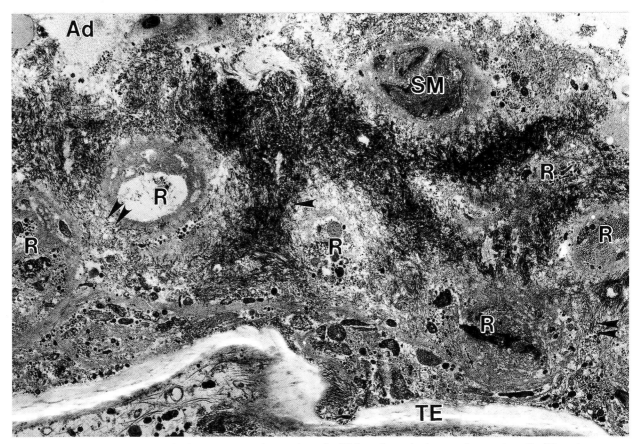

Figure 16 Electron micrograph showing smooth muscle cells (SM) and residual smooth muscle cells (R) within a coat of fibrillar (small arrow) and non-fibrillar (large arrows), partially degraded, Aβ. Ad, adventitia; TE, tunica elastica

mechanical properties of the vascular wall and to hemorrhage[44,45]. Smooth muscle cell-related β-amyloidosis appears in almost the entire cerebellar leptomeningeal network in PS1 mutation (P117L), indicating that amyloid production by smooth muscle cells might be enhanced by PS1 protein pathology[15].

β-Amyloid-related activation of glial cells

Microglial cell activation

Alzheimer-type pathology with β-amyloidosis and neurofibrillary pathology change the environment of the brain, and the interneuronal and interglial interactions. In the brain of patients with AD, there are approximately 40 proteins associated with the immune reaction; these include the classical complement cascade, complement inhibitors, acute-phase reactants, inflammatory cytokines, proteases and protease inhibitors, produced by activated astrocytes, microglial cells and neurons[46,47].

Microglial cells belong to the monocyte / macrophage system and play a major role in the immune response of the brain. Microglia are activated by numerous factors, including complement proteins[48] and Aβ[49]. Respiratory burst activity of microglial cells is associated with the production of superoxide anions and hydroxyl radicals, singlet oxygen species and hydrogen peroxide, which is necessary for phagocytic activity. In AD, activated microglial cells also release other compounds that are toxic to neurons, specifically, glutamate, tumor necrosis factor-α and nitric oxide[50,51]. The classical complement cascade is associated with the release of proteins that mark structures for opsonization and anaphyloxins that activate the membrane attack complex. Membrane attack complex inserts are detectable in the cell membrane in dystrophic neurites in classical plaques, but not in diffuse amyloid deposits[46,47]. The presence of these inserts and the release of numerous toxins by microglial cells may explain the selective edema of segments of neuronal processes in the plaque perimeter, and the accumulation of abnormal mitochondria, dense bodies and fibrils in the cytoskeleton.

Interleukin (IL)-1 of microglial origin activates astrocytes and contributes to astrocytosis[52]. Activated microglial cells of neuritic plaques overexpress acute-phase cytokine IL-1, which upregulates the expression and processing of AβPP with β-amyloid deposition[53]. Microglial IL-1 induces expression of protease inhibitor α_1-antichymotrypsin, thromboplastin, complement protein C and apo E, all of which are present in neuritic plaques. α_1-Antichymotrypsin acts as a chaperone protein[4,54], binding to β protein and promoting its polymerization into amyloid filaments[55]. Microglial cells and astrocytes produce apo E[56,57], which interacts with both normal soluble Aβ and fibrillar amyloid in plaques[58].

Extracellular Aβ upregulates amyloidogenic processing of βPP[59,60] through the cellular receptor for Aβ[61,62]. Cultured microglial cells treated with Aβ enhance the secretion of IL-1[63] and basic fibroblast growth factor (bFGF), and proliferate. Both factors increase the synthesis of AβPP. A small amount of extracellular Aβ may activate this cascade and contribute to plaque development[63].

Astrocyte activation

Astrocytes produce apo E[56,57], IL-1[64,65], endothelin-1[66] and prostaglandin E[67]. Astrocyte functional status is partially dependent on microglial cells. IL-1 of microglial origin may contribute to astrocytosis and astrocytic activation, with overexpression of the astrocyte-derived cytokine S-100-β, which increases the level of intraneuronal free calcium, leading to neuronal degeneration and death[52,68]. Astrocyte proliferation, cellular hypertrophy and increased glial fibrillary acidic protein (GFAP) expression is a common feature of cerebral aging; however, in AD, the numerical density of astrocytes increases several times in comparison to age-matched control brains[69,70]. Astrocyte activation is associated with fibrillar Aβ-positive plaques, ghost tangles, amyloid-positive capillaries and ischemic neurons. The morphology of activated astrocytes suggests that their role in each of these pathological processes is different and lesion-specific.

The absence of activated astrocytes in diffuse non-fibrillar plaques of neuronal origin and activation of astrocytes in neuritic fibrilized plaques of microglial origin indicate that an astrocytic reaction is related mainly to extracellular fibrillar Aβ deposition. Electron microscopy shows that astrocytic processes proliferate in the plaque periphery, penetrate into Aβ deposits, isolate aggregates of fibrillar amyloid and divide large amyloid clusters into small wisps (Figure 17). Transformation of the fib-

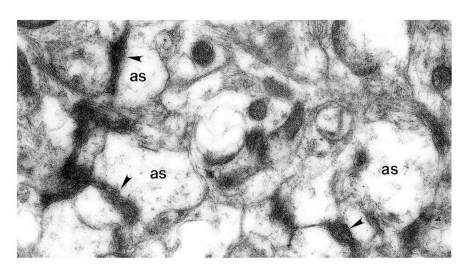

Figure 17 Electron micrograph showing wisps of partially degraded Aβ (arrowed) isolated between proliferating astrocytic processes (as) in the periphery of a neuritic plaque

rillar amyloid in the floccular or amorphous material lying between astrocytic processes indicates that astrocytic enzymes degrade amyloid fibrils[71].

The astrocytic reaction around amyloid deposits in the wall of obliterated capillaries recalls the astrocytic response to Aβ seen in neuritic plaques. Proliferating processes of activated astrocytes surround and degrade amyloid deposits. The absence of cell debris in the vascular wall, but the presence of well-preserved vascular amyloid hemistars, indicates that degradation of amyloid is much slower than degradation and removal of cells and cell debris.

Astrocytes are engaged in degradation and removal of neurons with neurofibrillary changes. In AD, in susceptible neuronal populations, abnormally phosphorylated tau accumulates, inhibiting microtubule assembly and disrupting preformed microtubules. Abnormally phosphorylated tau is the major protein subunit of paired helical filaments (PHF) of neurofibrillay tangles. After 3–4 years of degeneration with PHF accumulation, neurons die[72]. Cell debris and bundles of PHF losing their helical structure are penetrated by astrocytic processes. The fibrillar component is relatively resistant to degradation; however, a diminishing PHF component in the scar-like aggregates of cell residues and astrocytic processes indicates that degradation is effective (Figure 18). The prevalence of ghost tangles in brain structures such as sector CA1 of the horn of Ammon suggests that they remain in the tissue for a long time.

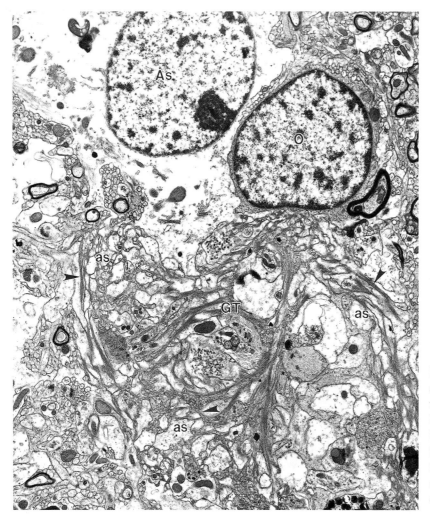

Figure 18 Electron micrograph showing ghost tangle (GT) degradation by an activated astrocyte (As). Residual PHFs are separated by proliferating astrocytic processes (as) into bundles and wisps, and degraded into straight filaments and amorphous material (arrowed). O, oligodendrocyte

Multifocal obliteration of capillaries causes regional ischemic changes with neuronal degeneration and death[41,42], and astrocyte proliferation and activation. Numerous swollen astrocytic processes intertwine with the shrunken bodies of ischemic neurons and degrade.

In the brain of patients with AD, the number of endothelin-1-immunoreactive astrocytes increases markedly in the periphery of plaques[66]. Endothelin-1 is a potent and long-lasting vasoconstrictor peptide[73], and its secretion by reactive astrocytes may induce constriction of arterioles and contribute to the local reduction of blood flow[74,75].

Astrocyte degeneration

In AD, astrocyte proliferation and activation is seen together with several forms of astrocyte degeneration, including cytoplasmic accumulation of PHFs, Rosenthal fibers, anchorage densities with desmosome-like structures, eosinophilic inclusions and corpora amylacea[76]. The appearance of tau-positive twisted and non-twisted tubules in astrocytes and oligodendrocytes[77,78] in AD, progressive supranuclear palsy[79] and Pick's disease suggests that an insult similar to that affecting neurons also affects glial cells and induces a similar response. Tau-positive fibrils share phosphorylation characteristics irrespective of the disease or cell type[80].

Rosenthal fibers develop in the brain with chronic reactive gliosis. The cause of Rosenthal fiber forma-tion might be overproduction or incomplete degradation of glial filaments[81]. In AD, Rosenthal fiber formation may be related to the involvement of astrocytes in the degradation and disposal of Aβ, PHF and neuronal debris during the chronic course of the disease[76].

Anchorage densities associated with hemidesmosome-like structures selectively reinforce perivascular astrocyte cell membrane facing the perivascular space. The development of these astrocytic changes in brains with atrophy of different origins[82], including AD[76], suggests that anchorage densities represent a non-specific reaction of astrocytes to brain atrophy.

In astrocytic eosinophilic inclusions[83], electron-dense granular or floccular material and the remnants of cytoplasmic organelles are detectable. The presence of fragments of rough endoplasmic reticulum and clusters of ribosomes embedded in electron-dense granular or floccular material indicates that, in AD, some astrocytes degenerate along with local non-lysosomal degradation of cytoplasmic components.

β-Amyloidosis is a part of the AD-specific cascade of pathological changes which leads, together with neurofibrillary changes, to neuronal degeneration and death, and functional deterioration.

References

1. Goldgaber D, Lerman MJ, McBride OW, et al. Characterization and chromosomal localization of a cDNA encoding brain amyloid of Alzheimer's disease. *Science* 1987;235:877–84

2. Kirschner DA, Inouye H, Duffy LK, et al. Synthetic peptide homologous to β protein from Alzheimer's disease forms amyloid-like fibrils *in vitro*. *Proc Natl Acad Sci USA* 1987;84:6953–7

3. Abraham CR, Selkoe DJ, Potter H. Immunochemical identification of the serine protease inhibitor α₁-antichymotrypsin in the brain amyloid deposits of Alzheimer's disease. *Cell* 1988;52:487–501

4. Picken MM, Larrondo-Lillo M, Coria F, et al. Distribution of the protease inhibitor α_1-antichymotrypsin in cerebral and systemic amyloid. *J Neuropathol Exp Neurol* 1990;49:41–8

5. Wisniewski HM, Vorbrodt AW, Wegiel J, et al. Ultrastructure of the cells forming amyloid fibers in Alzheimer's disease and scrapie. *Am J Med Genet* 1990;(Suppl 7):287–97

6. Snow AD, Mar H, Nochlin D, et al. The presence of heparan sulfate proteoglycans in the neuritic plaques and congophilic angiopathy in Alzheimer's disease. Am J Pathol 1988;133:456–63

7. Snow AD, Mar H, Nochlin D, et al. Early accumulation of heparan sulfate in neurons and in the beta-amyloid protein containing lesions of Alzheimer's disease and Down's syndrome. Am J Pathol 1990; 137:1253–70

8. Castano EM, Frangione B. Biology of disease: Human amyloidosis, Alzheimer's disease and related disorders. Lab Invest 1988;58:122–32

9. Coria F, Castano E, Prelli F, et al. Isolation and characterization of amyloid P-component from Alzheimer's disease and other cerebral amyloidosis. Lab Invest 1998;58:454–8

10. Schmechel DE, Saunders AM, Strittmatter WJ, et al. Increased amyloid β-deposition as a consequence of apolipoprotein E genotype in late-onset Alzheimer's disease. Proc Natl Acad Sci USA 1993;90:9649–53

11. Strittmatter WJ, Weisgraber KH, Huang DY, et al. Binding of human apolipoprotein E to synthetic amyloid β peptide: Isoform specific effects and implications for late-onset Alzheimer's disease. Proc Natl Acad Sci USA 1993;90:8098–102

12. Teller JK, Russo C, DeBusk LM, et al. Presence of soluble amyloid β-peptide precedes amyloid plaque formation in Down's syndrome. Nature Med 1996; 2:93–5

13. Wisniewski HM, Wegiel J, Popovitch ER. Age-associated development of diffuse and thioflavine-S-positive plaques in Down's syndrome. Dev Brain Dysfunct 1994;7:330–9

14. Gomez-Isla T, Wasco W, Pettingell WP, et al. A novel presenilin-1 mutation: Increased β-amyloid and neurofibrillary changes. Ann Neurol 1997;41:809–13

15. Wegiel J, Wisniewski HM, Kuchna I, et al. Cell-type-specific enhancement of β-amyloid deposition in a novel presenilin-1 mutation (P117L). J Neuropathol Exp Neurol 1998;57:831–8

16. Rebeck GW, Reiter JS, Stickland DK, et al. Apolipoprotein E in sporadic Alzheimer's disease: Allelic variation and receptor interactions. Neuron 1993;11: 575–80

17. Games D, Adams D, Alessandrini R, et al. Alzheimer-type neuropathology in transgenic mice overexpressing V717F beta-amyloid precursor protein. Nature 1995;373:523–7

18. Hsiao K, Chapman P, Nilsen S. Correlative memory deficits, Aβ elevation, and amyloid plaques in transgenic mice. Science 1996;274:99–102

19. Masliah E, Sisk A, Mallory M, et al. Comparison of neurodegenerative pathology in transgenic mice overexpressing V717F beta-amyloid precursor protein and Alzheimer's disease. J Neurosci 1996;16: 5795–811

20. Sturchler-Pierrat C, Abramowski D, Duke M, et al. Two amyloid precursor protein transgenic mice models with Alzheimer's disease-like pathology. Proc Natl Acad Sci USA 1997;94:13287–92

21. LaFeria FM, Hall CK, Ngo L, et al. Extracellular deposition of beta-amyloid upon p53-dependent neuronal cell death in transgenic mice. J Clin Invest 1996;98: 1626–32

22. Seubert P, Vigo-Pelfrey C, Esch F, et al. Isolation and quantification of soluble Alzheimer's β-peptide from biological fluids. Nature 1992;359:325–7

23. Frackowiak J, Mazur-Kolecka B, Wisniewski HM, et al. Secretion and accumulation of Alzheimer's β-protein by cultured vascular smooth muscle cells from old and young dogs. Brain Res 1995;676:225–30

24. Haass C, Schlossmacher M, Hung A, et al. Amyloid β-peptide is produced by cultured cells during normal metabolism. Nature 1992;359:322–5

25. Wisniewski HM, Wegiel J, Kotula L. Some neuropathological aspects of Alzheimer's disease and its relevance to other disciplines. Neuropathol Appl Neurobiol 1996;22:3–11

26. Cork LC, Masters C, Beyreuther K, et al. Development of senile plaques. Relationships of neuronal abnormalities and amyloid deposits. Am J Pathol 1990;137:1383–92

27. Li Y-T, Woodruff-Pak D, Trojanowski J. Amyloid plaques in cerebellar cortex and the integrity of Purkinje cell dendrites. Neurobiol Aging 1994;15:1–9

28. Pappolla MA, Omar RA, Vinters HV. Image analysis microspectroscopy shows that neurons participate in the genesis of a subset of early primitive (diffuse) senile plaques. *Am J Pathol* 1991;139:599–607

29. Probst A, Langui D, Ipsen S, *et al*. Deposition of beta/A4 protein along neuronal plasma membranes in diffuse senile plaques. *Acta Neuropathol* 1991;83: 21–9

30. Wisniewski HM, Sadowski M, Jakubowska-Sadowska K, *et al*. Diffuse, lake-like β-amyloid deposits in the parvopyramidal layer of the presubiculum in Alzheimer's disease. *J Neuropathol Exp Neurol* 1998;57:674–83

31. Lalowski M, Golabek A, Lemere CA, *et al*. The non-amyloidogenic p3 fragment (amyloid beta 17–42) is a major constituent of Down's syndrome cerebellar preamyloid. *J Biol Chem* 1996;271:33623–31

32. Wisniewski HM, Terry RD. Reexamination of the pathogenesis of the senile plaque. In: Zimmerman HM, ed. *Progress in Neuropathology, Vol II*. New York: Grune and Stratton, 1973:1–16

33. Wegiel J, Wisniewski HM. The complex of micro-glial cells and amyloid star in three-dimensional reconstruction. *Acta Neuropathol* 1990;81:116–24

34. Wisniewski HM, Wegiel J, Wang K-C, *et al*. Ultrastructural studies of the cells forming amyloid fibers in classical plaques. *Can J Neurol Sci* 1989;16:535–42

35. Wegiel J, Wisniewski HM. Tubuloreticular structures in microglial cells, pericytes and endothelial cells in Alzheimer's disease. *Acta Neuropathol* 1992; 83:653–8

36. Werb Z, Takemura R, Stenberg PE, *et al*. Directed exocytosis of secretory granules containing apolipoprotein E to the adherent surface and basal vacuoles of macrophages spreading on immobile immune complexes. *Am J Pathol* 1989;134:661–70

37. Lawson LJ, Perry WH, Gordon S. Turnover of resident microglia in the normal adult mouse brain. *Neuroscience* 1992;48:405–15

38. Graeber MB, Streit WJ, Buringer D, *et al*. Ultra-structural localization of major histocompatibility complex (MHC) class II-positive perivascular cells in histologically normal human brain. *J Neuropathol Exp Neurol* 1992;51:303–11

39. Hickey WF, Kimura H. Perivascular microglial cells of the CNS are bone marrow-derived and present antigen *in vivo*. *Science* 1988;239:290–2

40. Hickey WF, Vass K, Lassman H. Bone-marrow-derived elements in the central nervous system: An immunohistochemical and ultrastructural survey of rat chimeras. *J Neuropathol Exp Neurol* 1992;51: 246–56

41. Wisniewski HM, Wegiel J, Wang K-C, *et al*. Ultra-structural studies of the cells forming amyloid in the vessel wall in Alzheimer's disease. *Acta Neuropathol* 1992;84:117–27

42. Wisniewski HM, Wegiel J. Migration of perivascular cells into the neuropil and their involvement in β-amyloid plaque formation. *Acta Neuropathol* 1993; 85:586–95

43. Wisniewski HM, Wegiel J. β-amyloid formation by myocytes of leptomeningeal vessels. *Acta Neuropathol* 1994:87:233–41

44. Mandybur TI, Stephen RD, Bates SRD. Fatal massive intracerebral hemorrhage complicating cerebral amyloid angiopathy. *Arch Neurol* 1978;35:246–8

45. Thorack RM. Congophilic angiopathy complicated by surgery and massive hemorrhage. *Am J Pathol* 1975;81:349–66

46. McGeer EG, McGeer PL. The inflammatory response system of brain: Implications for therapy of Alzheimer's and other neurodegenerative disease. *Brain Res Rev* 1995;21:195–218

47. McGeer EG, McGeer PL. Inflammation in the brain in Alzheimer's disease: Implications for therapy. *Neuro Science News* 1998;1:29–35

48. Klegeris A, McGeer PL. Inhibition of respiratory burst in macrophages by complement receptor blockade. *Eur J Pharmacol* 1994;260:273–7

49. Klegeris A, Walker DG, McGeer PL. Activation of macrophages by Alzheimer β amyloid peptide. *Biochem Biophys Res Commun* 1994;199:984–1

50. Boje KM, Arora PK. Microglial-produced nitric oxide and reactive nitrogen oxides mediate neuronal cell death. *Brain Res* 1992;587:250–6

51. Chao CC, Hu S, Molitor TW, et al. Activated microglia mediate neuronal cell injury via a nitric oxide mechanism. J Immunol 1992;149:2736–41

52. Giulian D, Lachman LB. Interleukin-1 stimulation of astroglial proliferation after brain injury. Science 1985;228:497–9

53. Sheng JG, Ito K, Skinner RD, et al. In vivo and in vitro evidence supporting a role for the inflammatory cytokine interleukin-1 as a driving force in Alzheimer pathogenesis. Neurobiol Aging 1996;17:761–6

54. Potter H, Abraham CR, Dressler D. The Alzheimer amyloid components α_1-antichymotrypsin and β-protein form a stable complex in vitro. In: Iqbal K, McLachlan DRC, Winblad B, et al., eds. Alzheimer's Disease. Chichester: John Wiley and Sons Ltd, 1991: 275–9

55. Das S, Potter H. Expression of the Alzheimer amyloid-promoting factor antichymotrypsin is induced in human astrocytes by IL-1. Neuron 1995;14:447–56

56. Pitas RE, Boyle JK, Lee SH, et al. Astrocytes synthesize apolipoprotein E and metabolize apolipoprotein E-containing lipoproteins. Biochem Biophys Acta 1987; 917:148–61

57. Poirier J, Hess M, May PC, et al. Astrocytic apolipoprotein E mRNA and GFAP mRNA in hippocampus after entorhinal cortex lesioning. Mol Brain Res 1991;11:97–106

58. Wisniewski T, Golabek A, Matsubara E, et al. Apolipoprotein E: Binding to soluble Alzheimer's β-amyloid. Biochem Biophys Res Commun 1993;192:359–65

59. Davis-Salinas J, Saporito-Irvin SM, Cotman CW, et al. Amyloid β-protein induces its own production in cultured degenerating cerebrovascular smooth muscle cells. J Neurochem 1995;65:931–4

60. Yang AJ, Knauer M, Burdick DA, et al. Intracellular $A\beta 1$–42 aggregates stimulate the accumulation of stable, insoluble amyloidogenic fragments of the amyloid precursor protein in transfected cells. J Biol Chem 1995;270:14786–92

61. Khoury EJ, Hickman SE, Thomas CA, et al. Scavenger receptor-mediated adhesion of microglia to β-amyloid fibrils. Nature 1996;382:716–9

62. Yan SD, Chen X, Fu J, et al. RAGE and amyloid-β peptide neurotoxicity in Alzheimer's disease. Nature 1996;382:685–91

63. Araujo DM, Cotman CW. Beta-amyloid stimulates glial cells in vitro to produce growth factors that accumulate in senile plaques in Alzheimer's disease. Brain Res 1992;569;141–5

64. Bakhit C, Armanini M, Bennett GL, et al. Increase in glia-derived nerve growth factor following destruction of hippocampal neurons. Brain Res 1991;560: 76–83

65. Fonatana A, Kristensen F, Dubs R, et al. Production of prostaglandin E and an interleukin-1-like factor by cultured astrocytes and C6 glioma cells. J Immunol 1982;129:2413–9

66. Zhang WW, Badonic T, Höög A, et al. Astrocytes in Alzheimer's disease express immunoreactivity to the vasoconstrictor endothelin-1. J Neurol Sci 1994; 122:90–6

67. Akiyama H, Kawamata T, Yamada T, et al. Expression of intercellular adhesion molecule (ICAM)-1 by a subset of astrocytes in Alzheimer's disease and some other degenerative neurological disorders. Acta Neuropathol 1993;85:628–34

68. Gray CW, Patel AJ. Regulation of beta-amyloid precursor protein isoform mRNAs by transforming growth factor-beta 1 and interleukin-1 beta in astrocytes. Brain Res Mol 1993;19:251–6

69. Delacourte A. General and dramatic glial reaction in Alzheimer brains. Neurology 1990;40:33–7

70. Schechter R, Yen SHC, Terry RD. Fibrous astrocytes in senile dementia of Alzheimer type. J Neuropathol Exp Neurol 1981;40:95–101

71. Wisniewski HM, Wegiel J. Spatial relationships between astrocytes and classical plaque components. Neurobiol Aging 1991;12:593–600

72. Bobinski M, Wegiel J, Tarnawski M, et al. Duration of neurofibrillary changes in the hippocampal pyramidal neurons. Brain Res 1998;199:156–8

73. Lee M-E, Monte SMDL, Ng S-C, et al. Expression of the potent vasoconstrictor endothelin in the human central nervous system. J Clin Invest 1990; 86:141–7

74. Bonte FJ, Tintner R, Weiner MF, et al. Brain blood flow in the dementias: SPECT with histopathologic correlation. Radiology 1993;186;361–5

75. O'Brien JT, Eagger S, Syed GMS, et al. A study of regional cerebral blood flow and cognitive performance in Alzheimer's disease. J Neurol Neurosurg Psychiatr 1992;55:1182–7

76. Wegiel J, Wisniewski HM. Rosenthal fibers, eosinophilic inclusions, and anchorage densities with desmosome-like structures in astrocytes in Alzheimer's disease. Acta Neuropathol 1993;87:355–61

77. Nishimura M, Namba Y, Ikeda K. et al. Glial fibrillary tangles with straight tubules in the brains of patients with progressive supranuclear palsy. Neurosci Lett 1992;143:35–8

78. Nishimura M, Tomimoto H, Suenaga T, et al. Immunocytochemical characterization of glial fibrillary tangles in Alzheimer's disease brain. Am J Pathol 1995;146:1052–8

79. Yamada T, Calne DB, Akiyama H, et al. Further observations on tau-positive glia in the brains with progressive supranuclear palsy. Acta Neuropathol 1993;85:308–15

80. Iwatsubo T, Hasegawa M, Ihara Y. Neuronal and glial tau-positive inclusions in diverse neurologic diseases share common phosphorylation characteristics. Acta Neuropathol 1994;88:129–36

81. Goldman JE, Corbin E. Isolation of major protein component of Rosenthal fibers. Am J Pathol 1988; 130:569–78

82. Nakano I, Kato S, Yazawa I, et al. Anchorage densities associated with hemidesmosome-like structures in perivascular reactive astrocytes. Acta Neuropathol 1992;84:85–8

83. Abe H, Yagashita S, Itoh K, et al. Novel eosinophilic inclusion in astrocytes. Acta Neuropathol 1992;83: 659–63

8 Amyloid: chemical and molecular considerations

Thomas Wisniewski and Blas Frangione

Introduction

Degenerative diseases are becoming increasingly important causes of morbidity and mortality as the aged population in the Western world grows more numerous. Many of these disorders are now recognized to be related to abnormalities in protein conformation (Table 1). A paramount theme in the pathogenesis of these diseases is the conversion of a soluble normal protein into an insoluble, aggregated, β-sheet-rich form that, over time, leads to disease.

The prototype of these disorders are the amyloidoses. The most common amyloidosis occurs in Alzheimer's disease, in which a central event is the conversion of the normal soluble β-amyloid (sAβ) peptide to β-amyloid (Aβ) within neuritic plaques and cerebral vessels, where it is associated with toxicity[1] (Figure 1).

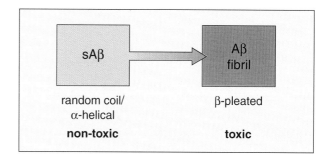

Figure 1 Possible change in AD of normal soluble β-amyloid (sAβ) peptide conformation to the β-amyloid (Aβ) deposited in plaques and in congophilic angiopathy

Table 1 Neurogenerative disease characterized by abnormal protein structure

Disease	Protein	Normal structure	Abnormal structure	Site of accumulation
AD	β-amyloid	α helix and random coil	β-pleated	extracellular (amyloid)
Prionosis	PrP	α helix and random coil	β-pleated	extracellular (amyloid)
Huntington's	huntingtin	< 35 CAG repeats	> 36 CAG repeats	nuclear
Parkinson's	α-synuclein	soluble	aggregated	cytoplasmic
SCA (1–3, 7)	ataxin	few CAG repeats	many CAG repeats	nuclear
DRPLA	atrophin-1	< 36 CAG repeats	> 49 CAG repeats	nuclear
SBMA	androgen	< 36 CAG repeats	> 38 CAG repeats	nuclear

SCA, spinocerebellar ataxia; DRPLA, dentatorubropallidoluysial atrophy; SBMA, spinobulbar muscular atrophy

Recently, another group of neurodegenerative disorders, marked by trinucleotide (CAG) repeats, and including Huntington's disease and spinocerebellar ataxia, has been recognized (see Table 1)[2,3]. These trinucleotide repeats lead to insertions of increasing lengths of glutamine within the protein, thereby increasing the tendency of the protein to aggregate and form intracellular neuronal inclusions leading to cell death.

From a mechanistic point of view, the best understood of the conformational disorders are the prion-related diseases (or prionoses). The etiology of these diseases is the conversion of the normal prion protein PrP^C into the infectious and pathogenic form PrP^{Sc} [4,5]. PrP^C and PrP^{Sc} are thought to differ only in their conformation, with PrP^{Sc} having a greater β-sheet content. Abnormal protein folding is also a recognized hallmark of normal aging[6].

These diseases all involve the accumulation of protein with an abnormal conformation, a process which is also promoted by the presence of mutations in particular gene products and chaperone proteins. Thus, protein conformational disorders may be regarded as part of an aberrant aging process that is influenced by genetic factors.

Alzheimer's disease (AD) is the most common cause of late-life dementia[6]. AD may be divided into an early-onset (<60 years of age) form and a more common late-onset (>60 years of age) form. So far, three genes have been linked to early-onset AD: the β-amyloid precursor protein (βPP) on chromosome 21[7,8]; presenilin 1 (PS1) on chromosome 14[9,10]; and presenilin 2 (PS2) on chromosome 1[11–13]. The majority of cases of early-onset AD is thought to be related to mutations in PS1 and PS2 whereas, in late-onset AD, an association with the inheritance of the apolipoprotein E (apo E) allele E4 has been described[14,15].

The presence of the apo E4 allele appears to be a predominant risk factor for patients with onset of AD at 60–70 years of age[16]. Apo E4 is also a risk factor for the related congophilic angiopathy[17,18] as well as multi-infarction dementia[19,20].

In terms of neuropathology, each of these subtypes of AD is characterized by four major lesions:

(1) Intraneuronal cytoplasmic deposits of neurofibrillary tangles (NFTs);

(2) Parenchymal amyloid deposits called neuritic plaques;

(3) Cerebrovascular amyloidosis; and

(4) Synaptic loss.

The major constituent of the neuritic plaques and congophilic angiopathy is Aβ, although these deposits also contain other proteins such as glycosaminoglycans and apolipoproteins[6]. Each of the proteins with linkage to AD have now been found to be components of neuritic plaques[21–23]. It remains to be determined whether all of these proteins are involved in the same or different pathological pathway(s), and which of these proteins is the most important for the most common, late-onset form of AD.

β-Amyloid protein expression

Aβ is a 39–44 amino-acid peptide that is heterogeneous at both its amino and carboxyl termini[21,24–27]. The amino-terminal sequence of this peptide was first determined by the seminal work of Dr G. Glenner in 1984[28]. Neuritic plaque amyloid was first sequenced in 1985[21] and was found to extend mainly to Aβ residue 42 / 43. Vascular amyloid was initially reported as Aβ 1–28[28], but was later found to extend mainly to Aβ 1–39 / 40[24,25].

This heterogeneity at the carboxyl terminus of Aβ was attributed to differences in local tissue processing. More recent reports, using different techniques, have also found Aβ 1–42 in vascular amyloid deposits[29]. The Aβ peptide is found at low concentrations as a normal constituent of biological fluids, where it is known as sAβ[30–33]. sAβ is predominantly Aβ 1–40, although shorter and longer sequences are found, including Aβ 1–28 and Aβ 1–42[34]. As the amino-acid sequence of sAβ is similar or identical to Aβ, it is likely that amyloid in AD is at least partially derived from sAβ from either the brain or a systemic source. Thus, one of the important issues in AD research is the identification of the factors involved in the conformational change of normal sAβ into the Aβ found in AD lesions (see Figure 1).

Both Aβ and sAβ are degradative fragments from a larger amyloid precursor protein (βPP)[35-38] (Figure 2). The βPP gene is located on chromosome 21 and contains at least 19 exons, spanning 400 kb of DNA; more then ten isoforms of βPP mRNA may be generated by alternative splicing[39-43]. The four major Aβ-containing products are proteins of 695, 714, 751 and 770 amino acids. The βPP has a predicted structure of a multidomain transmembrane cell surface receptor[35-38] (see Figure 2). The Aβ sequence arises from portions of exons 16 and 17; therefore, Aβ cannot be generated by alternative

splicing of βPP, and requires proteolytic cleavage at both its N and C termini.

One of the first metabolic processing pathways of βPP to be discovered involves a cleavage at Aβ residue 16 by the so-called α-secretase, which releases a large soluble protein containing only the N-terminal sequence of Aβ[44-47]. There are two other secretases, β-secretase and γ-secretase, thought to cleave βPP at the N and C termini, respectively, of the Aβ peptide (Figure 3).

With the discovery of sAβ, it became clear that an increased production of Aβ peptides from βPP is not a necessary component of the pathology of AD. Other events, such as tissue clearance of Aβ peptides and their conformation, may be critical in determining their local build-up and deposition in the AD brain.

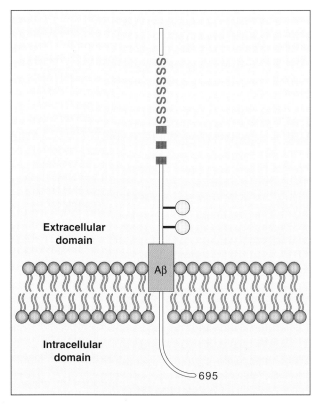

Figure 2 β-Amyloid precursor protein (βPP). Most of the protein is in the extracellular domain. The Aβ part (green) is partly extracellular and partly within the membrane. The cysteine-rich domain is blue;. an acidic domain is pink. The two glycosylation sites are yellow

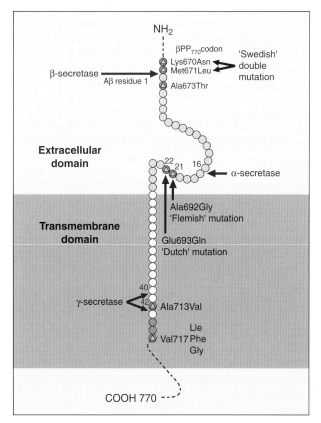

Figure 3 Aβ protein of βPP showing the mutations associated with FAD (red), the codon involved and the amino-acid substitution as well as the sites of cleavage by α-, β- and γ- secretases

Amyloid precursor protein mutations

A small subset of patients with early-onset (<55 years of age) familial AD (FAD) have been shown to be linked to a number of different mutations in the βPP gene (Table 2; see also Figure 3). The first βPP mutation described is seen among families with hereditary cerebral hemorrhage with amyloidosis, Dutch type (HCHWA-D)[7]. The pathology of this condition is characterized by the deposition of amyloid mainly in the cerebral vessels, with a halo of Aβ immunoreactivity in the parenchyma circumscribing many of the vessels[48]. This heavy Aβ deposition in cerebral vessels leads to strokes as a major clinical symptom. HCHWA-D is associated with a glutamine substitution for glutamic acid at codon 693 (βPP$_{770}$ numbering), corresponding to residue 22 of Aβ[7] (see Figure 3). A number of studies *in vitro* have shown that Aβ peptides containing this mutation have a greater fibrilogenic potential with a greater proportion in the Aβ_{ac} state[49–51] (Figure 4).

Other studies *in vitro* have provided a possible indication of how some of the other FAD mutations are associated with AD (Figure 5). Tissue culture studies have shown that cells transfected with the 'Swedish' double mutation at codons 670 / 671 secrete higher levels of sAβ peptides compared with cells expressing wild-type constructs[52,53]. On the other hand, cells expressing βPP mutations found at codon 717 do not appear to secrete higher total levels of sAβ, but produce a higher proportion of the longer, more hydrophobic, Aβ peptides that extend to residue 42[54]. The latter observation and other findings *in vitro* have led to the suggestion that the major pathogenic Aβ peptide may be Aβ 1–42, and that amyloid formation may be initiated by the presence of this longer and more fibrilogenic peptide[55,56].

Presenilins and Alzheimer's disease

Although mutations in the βPP gene were the first to be linked to FAD, it appears that these mutations are rare. Of the approximately 5% of cases of AD which has early onset and autosomal-dominant inheritance, only 1–3% is related to βPP mutations (Figure 6). It appears that 50–60% of FAD is linked to mutations of the PS1 and PS2 genes. A further locus linked to FAD has been found on chromosome 12; however, the gene has not yet been identified[3]. The PS1 gene on chromosome 14 was identified using a positional cloning strategy[9,10] whereas the PS2 gene on chromosome 1 was found on the basis of its homology to PS1[11–13]. These two genes have 67% amino-acid identity. Thus far, more than

Table 2 Pathogenic mutations of β-amyloid precursor protein

Codon	Amino-acid substitution	Phenotype	Cases described	Reference
670/671	Lys–Met → Asn–Leu	AD	one Swedish family	136
673	Ala → Thr	–	one case of stroke and MI	137
692	Ala → Gly	AD + cerebral hemorrhage	one Dutch family	138
693	Glu → Gln	HCHWA-D	three Dutch families	7
	Glu → Gly	–	one case of AD	139
713	Ala → Val	–	one case of schizophrenia	140
	Ala → Thr	–	one case of AD and several controls	141
717	Val → Ile	AD	three English and two Japanese families	142
	Val → Phe	AD	one American family	143
	Val → Gly	AD	one English family	144

AD, Alzheimer's disease; HCHWA-D, hereditary cerebral hemorrhage with amyloidosis, Dutch type

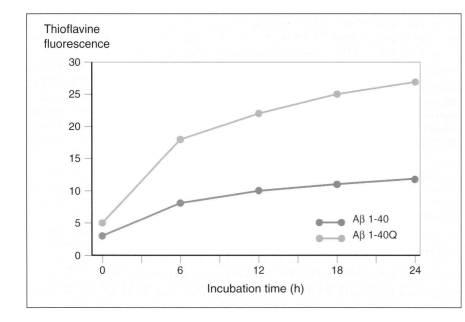

Figure 4 Fibril formation *in vitro* of wild-type Aβ 1–40 *vs* Aβ 1–40Q, which contains the mutation associated with HCHWA-D. The amount of thioflavine T fluorescence corresponds to the quantity of amyloid fibrils formed. Thus, Aβ peptides containing the Dutch mutation have a greater fibril-forming capability

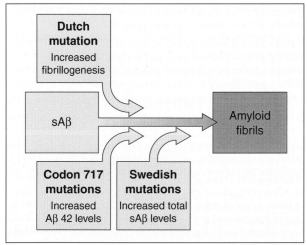

Figure 5 Proposed effects of the various mutations of βPP. Each mutation increases the conversion of sAβ to Aβ

Figure 6 Approximate proportions of early-onset FAD associated with the various gene mutations

46 mutations have been reported in PS1, and three have been found in PS2 among early-onset FAD pedigrees[57–59].

Recently, an additional PS1 mutation was found in a Polish FAD kindred of P117L[60,61]. This family illustrates the dramatic phenotype associated with many of the presenilin mutations. In this particular kindred, the onset of AD was as early as age 23 years, with death due to AD at age 28 years[60] (Figure 7). The amyloid burden among PS1-linked FAD patients also appears to be greatly

increased[61] (Figure 8). Because the neuropathological features of presenilin-linked FAD are similar to the more common late-onset form of AD, it is presumed that understanding the role of presenilin in FAD will help to elucidate the pathology of all forms of AD.

The PS1 and PS2 genes encode predicted proteins of 467 and 448 amino acids, respectively, with numerous transmembrane domains[57] (Figure 9). Recent studies of PS1 topology have indicated the existence of either six or eight transmembrane domains with both amino and carboxyl termini located in the cytoplasm[62–64] (see Figure 7). The mRNA of both PS1 and PS2 has been found in many different tissues and cell lines, with high levels in the brain and neurons[10,65,66]. In the normal brain, immunohistochemical studies have shown the presence of presenilin predominantly in neuronal cells, where it is preferentially concentrated in the cytoplasm and dendrites[67–70]. These immunocytochemical studies have also suggested a predominant localization to the endoplasmic reticulum and Golgi complex[66,71].

Investigations of PS1 processing in cell lines and brain tissue have shown that a portion of PS1 undergoes endoproteolytic cleavage to at least two major fragments: a 17 kDa carboxyl-terminal fragment; and a ~27 kDa amino-terminal fragment[72] (Figure 9).

The normal biological role of these proteins remains unknown; however, clues may be found in the known functions of two *Caenorhabditis elegans* proteins with which presenilins are homologous, namely, sel-12 (50% identical to presenilin)[73] and

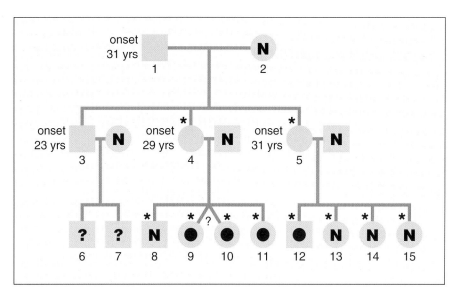

Figure 7 Polish pedigree with FAD associated with PS1 mutation (P117L), includes the age of AD symptom-onset among affected individuals. The patient with onset at age 23 years died due to AD at 28 years of age

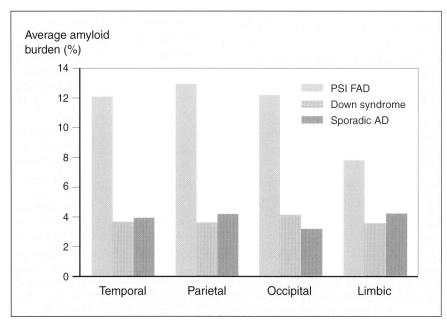

Figure 8 Amyloid burden in different regions of the brain among patients with the PS1 P117L mutation compared with patients with Down syndrome and sporadic AD (all patients were matched for the clinical stage of the disease)

spe-4 (25% homology to presenilin)[74]. More than 80% of the known FAD presenilin mutations occur in residues that are conserved in sel-12. This protein is known to be a facilitator of lin-12, a member of the Notch family of receptors involved with intercellular signaling associated with determining cell fate in the nematode[73]. Sel-12 may be a co-receptor for lin-12 or play a role in receptor trafficking and recycling. Such a role in cellular trafficking or protein processing is consistent with the proposed function for spe-4. Loss-of-function mutations in spe-4 disrupt the delivery of proteins to spermatids during spermatogenesis in the nematode[74].

Whatever the normal role of presenilin, it is clear from experiments with PS1 knockout mice that presenilin is important for CNS development[75]. In these studies, the knockout mice died during late gestation due to massive hemorrhage that was limited to the brain and spinal cord beneath the primordial dura and leptomeninges as well as within the ventricles and parenchyma of the brain[75]. Thus, loss of presenilin function does not appear to be compatible with life. The prominence of cerebral vessel pathology in these knockout mice is of interest as it is known that presenilin is present in both normal cerebral vessels and congophilic angiopathy[76,77].

How presenilin is involved in the pathogenesis of AD is unknown; however, there is some evidence to suggest a possible interaction with Aβ and / or βPP. Presenilin mutations influence the production of the more highly amyloidogenic 1–42 form of Aβ. This effect may be mediated by regulating γ-secretase activity[78]. Higher levels of Aβ 42 have been found in the plasma and cultured fibroblast media of PS1 and PS2 mutation carriers[79]. This increase has also been noted in the brain of transgenic mice and transfected cells[80–82]. Furthermore, immunohistochemical studies using antibodies for the carboxyl terminus of Aβ 42 have shown an increase of Aβ 42 deposits in the brain of AD patients with PS1 mutations[83], and transgenic mice coexpressing mutant βPP and PS1 proteins show accelerated amyloid deposition[84,85]. There are also reports that presenilin may be involved in programmed cell death (apoptosis). Expression of PS2 constructs has been shown to accelerate apoptosis in lymphocytes and PC12 cells[86,87], and expression of PS1 has been shown to sensitize PC12 and Jurkat cells to apoptotic stimuli[88,89].

Another piece of evidence suggesting interaction between presenilin and Aβ is the localization of presenilin epitopes within neuritic plaques. In 1995, we reported that an antibody raised to the carboxyl

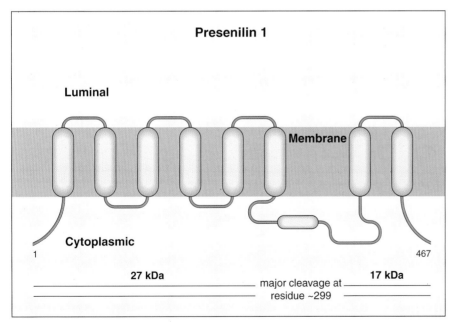

Figure 9 Proposed topology of PS1, which undergoes endoproteolytic cleavage to at least two major fragments: a 17 kDa carboxyl fragment; and a 27 kDa amino-terminal fragment

terminus of PS1 immunoreacted with some neuritic plaques[23] (Figure 10). This immunoreactivity was found in neuritic plaques of both PS1-linked FAD patients and in late-onset sporadic AD, suggesting a general role for presenilin in AD. Since then, additional reports using other antibodies have immunohistochemically confirmed the presence of presenilin in association with the amyloid of AD neuritic plaques[67,68,77,90].

The observation that antibodies raised to carboxyl epitopes of presenilin immunoreact with neuritic plaques has been confirmed biochemically[76]. It was found that the 17 kDa carboxyl fragment of presenilin was also present in partially purified neuritic plaque amyloid fractions and that this fragment appeared to bind to Aβ. The identity of this presenilin fragment was confirmed by amino-acid sequencing and found to begin at residue 300 (see Figure 9)[76]. This finding is similar to that of a study where the main cleavage site of PS1 was found to occur between residues 298–299 in cells transfected with human PS1[91]. These findings further support a possible close association between presenilin and Aβ / βPP. However, the role of presenilin in the pathogenesis of AD remains unclear.

Alzheimer's disease and apolipoprotein E

Our immunohistochemical studies and those of other researchers have identified apolipoprotein E (apo E) as an amyloid-associated protein found in AD plaque lesions (Figure 11)[92,93]. This immunohistochemical co-localization led us to propose that apo E may function as a 'pathological chaperone' in the pathogenesis of AD (Figure 12). In this context, the term refers to a protein that interacts with β-amyloid and helps to stabilize an abnormal intermediate conformation which is associated with disease (see Figure 12). This contrasts with normal physiological chaperone proteins, which induce the normal native protein conformation[94]. Since proposing this theory, it has become clear that inheritance of a particular allele of apo E (apo E4) is a major risk factor for late-onset AD[14,15]. In humans, the apo E gene is polymorphic, leading to three major apo E isoforms, namely, E2, E3 and E4. Apo E3, the most common isoform, has cysteine at position 112 and arginine at position 158; apo E2 is the least common isoform, with cysteine at both positions whereas apo E4 presents arginine at both sites[95]. Inheritance of the apo E4 allele is associated with an increased risk of late-onset sporadic AD.

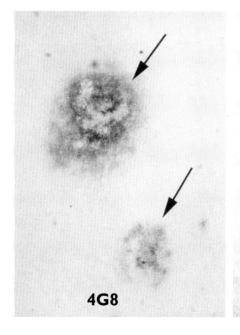
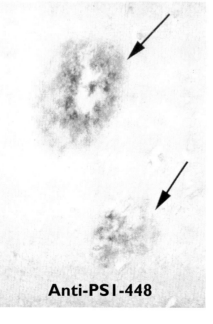

4G8 **Anti-PS1-448**

Figure 10 Immunohistochemical immunoreactivity of a neuritic plaque, using a monoclonal antibody to Aβ (4G8; left) and a polyclonal antibody to a carboxyl-terminal epitope of PS1 (right) to demonstrate the immunohistochemical localization of a PS1 epitope in some neuritic plaques

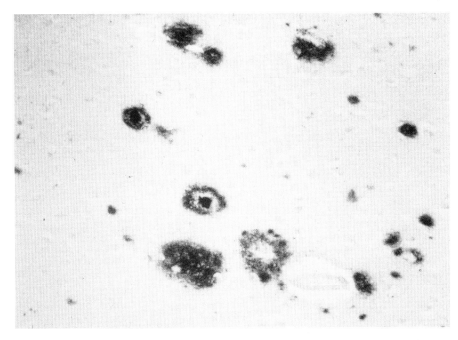

Figure 11 Immunohistochemically stained AD neuritic plaques using apo E antibody

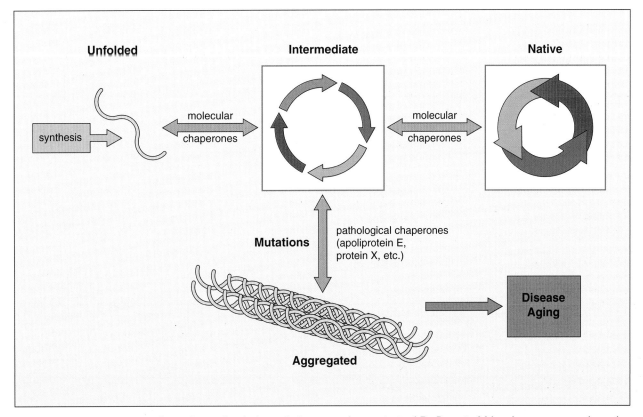

Figure 12 Potential role of apo E as a 'pathological chaperone' protein in AD. Protein X has been proposed to play a similar role in prion-related diseases

Studies of the linkage between apo E4 and AD have shown that:

(1) Carriers of the E4 allele have an increased risk of developing AD in an allelic dose-dependent manner;

(2) The apo E4 genotype modulates the age of onset of the disease[14,15]; and

(3) Inheritance of the E4 allele correlates with increased deposition of Aβ in blood vessels and plaques, and a greater density of senile plaques in the cerebral cortex[96,97].

The effect of apo E4 has been found to be of greatest significance among patients with an onset of disease at ages 60–70 years[16]. The apo E locus is not considered a causative gene, but rather a susceptibility or modifying factor as the presence of the E4 allele is neither sufficient nor necessary for AD to develop. The role of apo E in the pathogenesis of AD is unclear, and several possibilities have been proposed (Figure 13); however, there is considerable evidence to suggest a direct interaction between apo E and Aβ.

Apo E has been shown to bind Aβ peptides that have a high K_d, and preferentially binds Aβ peptides with a β-sheet conformation[98]. This interaction is likely to take place *in vivo* as it has been documented that a carboxyl fragment of apo E co-purifies with Aβ from neuritic plaques[22]. Amino-acid sequencing reveals that this fragment has a ragged amino terminus with starts corresponding to apo E residues 216 and 193[22]. Other researchers have also confirmed the presence of apo E and its fragments biochemically in neuritic plaques[99]. Furthermore, under certain conditions *in vitro*, apo E4 has been shown to promote more Aβ peptide fibrilogenesis than either apo E3 or E2[100–102] (Figure 14). Finally, the proposed role of apo E as a pathological chaperone protein is supported by recent transgenic mouse studies showing that, when apo E knockout mice are crossed with mice that overexpress mutated βPP and normally develop cerebral amyloid deposits with age, amyloid deposition was greatly reduced (Figure 15)[103].

Interactions between apo E and Aβ peptides may also influence the clearance of Aβ peptides from the brain (Figure 16). Experiments in a rat model showed that synthetic Aβ 1–40 is normally rapidly cleared from the brain[104]. It was found that following a brief infusion of ^{125}I-sAβ peptide into one lateral ventricle in a normal rat, 30% of the infusion was cleared from the ventricular CSF to the bloodstream by 3.5 min after administration; a further 30% was removed over the next 6.5 min[104]. These results suggest that clearance of sAβ pep-

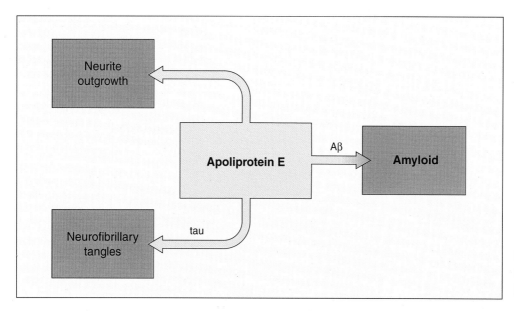

Figure 13 Potential roles of apo E in the pathogenesis of AD

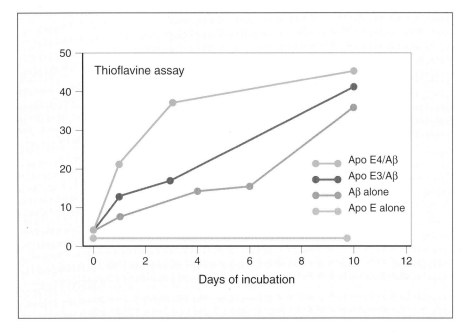

Figure 14 Under certain conditions *in vitro*, apo E promotes Aβ fibril formation, as shown by thioflavine T assay. In particular, apo E4 promotes fibril formation

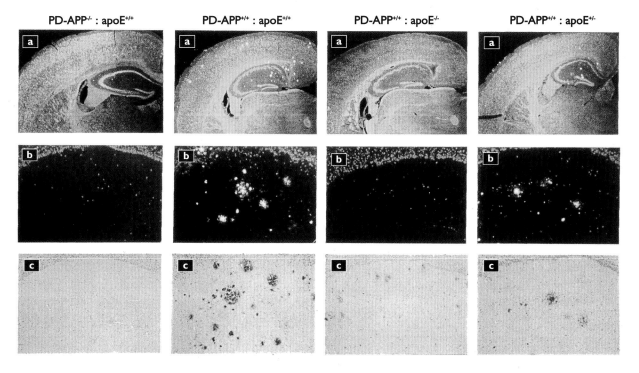

Figure 15 Lack of apo E dramatically reduces Aβ deposition in a transgenic mouse model of AD in which mutant βPP is overexpressed (PD-APP transgenic mice). In 6-month-old mice homozygous for the PD-APP transgene wild type for the mouse apo E gene (PD-APP⁺/⁺ apo E⁺/⁺; column B), numerous large thioflavine S-fluorescent (rows a and b) and Aβ-immunoreactive deposits (row c) are evident in the cerebral cortex (row a) and hippocampus (rows b and c). In contrast, in 6-month-old PD-APP⁺/⁺ apoE⁻/⁻ mice, no thioflavine S-fluorescent deposits were observed (column C). PD-APP⁺/⁺ apo E⁺/⁻ mice of the same age and gender had reduced (essentially intermediate) levels of thioflavine S-fluorescent and Aβ-immunoreactive deposits (column D). Column A shows controls (PD-APP⁻/⁻ apo E⁺/⁺). Reproduced from reference 103, with permission

tide across the blood–brain barrier (BBB) may be an important mechanism for regulation of brain sAβ levels. The presence of brain sAβ–apo E complexes has been shown to occur in the AD brain[105]. The involvement of apo E in the clearance of brain sAβ is consistent with a recent study where transgenic mice overexpressing mutant βPP were crossed with mice knocked out for murine apo E, but expressed either human apoE3 or E4. In this mouse model of AD, the presence of human apoE3 or E4 markedly suppressed Aβ deposition at 9 months of age[106]. However, it is known that the passage of apo E is limited across the BBB, as shown by data from liver-transplant patients. Following liver transplantation, the plasma apoE phenotype of the recipient changed to that of the liver donor; however, the apoE phenotype in the CSF does not changes, indicating that the brain apoE is synthesized locally[107]. We suggest that, in patients with the apoE4 allele, formation of brain sAβ–apoE4 complexes (as compared to sAβ–apoE3 or E2 complexes) can lead to both a reduced clearance of Aβ peptides, as well as a direct amyloid fibril promoting effect of apoE4 (see Figure 16).

Theories of the pathogenesis of Alzheimer's disease

According to many AD researchers, Aβ accumulation may be considered central to the pathogenesis of AD as it either directly or indirectly through a number of downstream events is 'causative' of the disease. This notion is part of the amyloid cascade hypothesis[108] (Figure 17). In current versions of this hypothesis, it is thought that Aβ peptides which extend to residue 42 (Aβ 42) are first deposited in preamyloid lesions (or diffuse plaques). These amorphous, irregularly bordered, roughly spherical areas are immunoreactive to anti-Aβ antibodies and associated with few or no dystrophic neurites. Preamyloid deposits, unlike amyloid, are not stained by Congo red or thioflavine S[109–113].

Extensive numbers of preamyloid lesions may be found in aged individuals with no reported clinical symptoms[114–116]. In Down syndrome patients, who have three copies of the βPP gene, preamyloid lesions may appear as early as age 12 years[117–119]. Over a period of years, these lesions are thought to

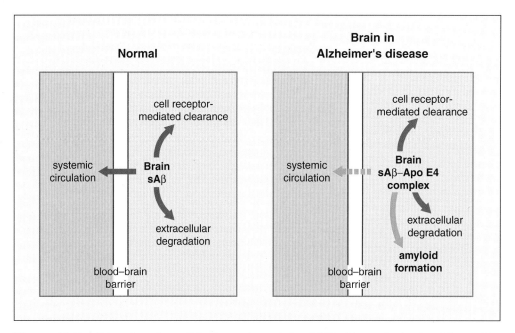

Figure 16 Possible roles of apo E in the pathogenesis of AD. Normally, brain sAβ peptides are rapidly cleared but, in AD, because of a rise in the levels of sAβ peptides and / or apo E, apo E–Aβ complexes are formed. In patients with the apo E4 allele, the sAβ–apoE4 complexes are clearly less effective than sAβ–apo E3 or E2 complexes. Thus, apo E4 may directly promote amyloid fibril formation as well as being less effective at clearing brain Aβ peptides, relative to apoE3 or E2

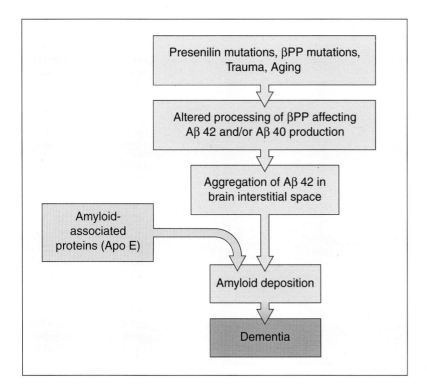

Figure 17 Amyloid cascade hypothesis. The diagram shows pathways leading to amyloid deposition, neuronal loss and the dementia of Alzheimer's disease

become compacted, at which point they acquire the characteristics of amyloid, and are associated with neuronal damage and NFTs in the form of neuritic plaques[108].

In addition to the above data, at least four other pieces of evidence have been used to substantiate the amyloid cascade hypothesis:

(1) Clinically, normal aged individuals may develop extensive preamyloid deposits which may herald the later development of AD pathology[120];

(2) Studies *in vitro* using Aβ synthetic peptides have shown that toxicity is dependent on the presence of a fibrillar, predominantly β-sheet conformation[121–125];

(3) As already discussed, some rare early-onset FAD pedigrees are linked to βPP mutations. Studies using transfected cells with the Swedish double mutation at codons 670 / 671 of βPP have shown that this leads to higher levels of total sAβ peptides compared with cells expressing wild-type con-

structs[52,53]. In contrast, cells expressing βPP mutations at codon 717 produce a higher proportion of the longer, more hydrophobic, Aβ peptides that extend to residue 42[54] (see Figure 7.3);

(4) Transgenic mice expressing high levels of mutant human βPP show the development of diffuse and amyloid plaques[126,127].

Alternative hypotheses for the pathogenesis of AD suggest that the deposition of Aβ in the form of amyloid is only a marker of a disease process that is not directly linked to the causation of dementia (Figure 18). Damaging evidence for the amyloid hypothesis comes from two transgenic mouse models of AD: the PD-APP mouse[126] and the PrP-APP mouse[127]. In both these models, despite extensive amyloid deposition, no significant neuronal loss has been detected[128,129]. In another transgenic mouse model, APP23 mice, which express APP with the Swedish FAD mutation, neuronal loss has been documented in the CA1 sector of the hippocampus, but not in the neocortex[130]. Despite some neuronal loss in the lattermost mouse model, these results remain problematic for the amyloid hypothesis as

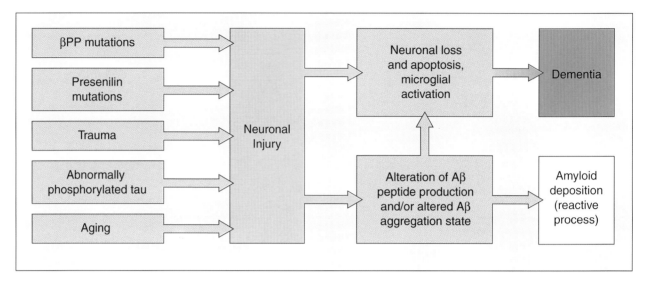

Figure 18 An alternative to the amyloid cascade hypothesis

they raise the question of why neuronal loss is not more prominent in these mouse models, given the observed extensive amyloid deposits.

These studies indicate that fibrillar deposits *per se* are not necessarily neurotoxic *in vivo*. Other co-depositing proteins may be necessary for the development of toxicity *in vivo* (such as certain amyloid-associated proteins and inflammatory factors). Additional difficulties for a strict interpretation of the amyloid hypothesis comes from studies of the levels of brain sAβ peptides in some of these transgenic models. Measurement of sAβ in different regions of the brain in homozygous transgenic mice[126], in which FAD mutant βPP is overexpressed, shows elevations even in areas such as the thalamus where amyloid deposition does not occur (or is rare)[131]. The sAβ levels in the thalamus of homozygous animals are essentially the same as sAβ levels in the hippocampus of heterozygous transgenic mice, where amyloid does occur. This indicates that a threshold concentration of sAβ is not sufficient for amyloid deposition and that other regional brain specific factors are also required[131].

A further important observation in this transgenic mouse model is the dramatic rise in brain sAβ levels with age[131]. A 17-fold increase is seen at ages 4–8 months and, by 18 months, is 500-fold greater than the 4-month level. Over the same time period,

there is no age-dependent change in βPP nor is there any evidence of age-dependent increased processing of βPP to sAβ (as indicated by measuring levels of βPP processed with the β-secretase clip site)[131].

If the age-associated rise in brain sAβ is not due to increased production, then an alternative explanation is that the clearance of brain sAβ is reduced with age, leading to increasing levels. Furthermore, a number of biochemical and immunohistochemical studies of Aβ peptide deposition in the form of preamyloid has suggested that these lesions do not necessarily progress to neuritic plaque formation and that other factors in addition to the presence of Aβ 1–42 may be important for neuritic plaque formation[132,133]. A further consideration now taken by amyloidologists is the finding that tau mutations may also be associated with neuronal loss and dementia[134,135], suggesting that tau cannot be ignored in the cascade of pathological changes.

The combined effect of the above findings is to suggest that amyloid formation is a reactive process and that the 'Aβ only' hypothesis for the etiology of AD may need to be replaced by a proposal for 'Aβ and something else'. It is now evident that abnormalities in a number of different genes and several different pathogenetic pathways may be involved in the production of a final common pathway of neuritic plaque formation in AD (Figure 19).

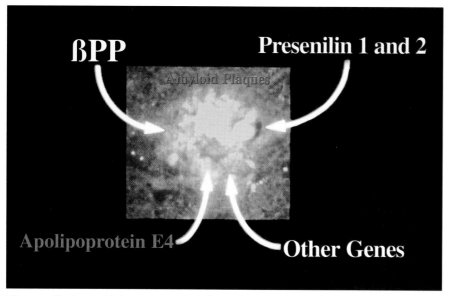

Figure 19 As multiple genes and pathways are involved in AD, it may be more appropriate to view AD as a syndrome rather than a single disease entity

Ultimately, it may become more appropriate to view AD as a syndrome rather than a single disease entity.

Acknowledgements

This work has been supported by NIH grants AG15408, AG08721 and AR02594.

References

1. Wisniewski T, Ghiso J, Frangione B. Biology of Aβ amyloid in Alzheimer's disease. *Neurobiol Dis* 1997; 4:313–28

2. Welch WJ, Gambetti P. Chaperoning brain diseases. *Nature* 1998;392:23–4

3. Pericak-Vance MA, Bass MP, Yamaoka LH, et al. Complete genomic screen in late-onset familial Alzheimer disease. Evidence for a new locus on chromosome 12. *J Am Med Assoc* 1997;278:1282–3

4. Prusiner SB, Scott MR, DeArmond SJ, et al. Prion protein biology. *Cell* 1998;93:337–48

5. Horwich AL, Weismann JS. Deadly conformations – protein misfolding in prion diseases. *Cell* 1997;89: 499–510

6. Wisniewski T, Frangione B. Molecular biology of brain aging and neurodegenerative disorders. *Acta Neurobiol Exp* 1996;56:267–79

7. Levy E, Carman MD, Fernandez-Madrid I, et al. Mutation of the Alzheimer's disease amyloid gene in hereditary cerebral hemorrhage, Dutch type. *Science* 1990;248:1124–6

8. Goate A, Chartier-Harlin M-C, Mullan M, et al. Segregation of a missense mutation in the amyloid precursor protein gene with familial Alzheimer's disease. *Nature* 1991;349:704–6

9. Schellenberg G. Genetic linkage for a novel familial Alzheimer's disease locus on chromosome 14. *Science* 1992;258:868–71

10. Sherrington R, Rogaev EI, Liang Y, et al. Cloning of a gene bearing missense mutations in early onset familial Alzheimer's disease. Nature 1995;375: 754–60

11. Levy-Lahad E, Wasco W, Poorkaj P, et al. Candidate gene for the chromosome 1 familial Alzheimer's disease locus. Science 1995;269:973–7

12. Rogaev E, Sherrington R, Rogaeva EA, et al. Familial Alzheimer's disease in kindreds with missense mutations in a gene on chromosome 1 related to the Alzheimer's disease type 3 gene. Nature 1995; 376:775–8

13. Li J, Ma J, Potter H. Identification and expression analysis of a potential familial Alzheimer disease gene on chromosome 1 related to AD3. Proc Natl Acad Sci (USA) 1995;92:12180–4

14. Corder EH, Saunders AM, Strittmatter WJ, et al. Gene dose of apolipoprotein E type 4 allele and the risk of Alzheimer's disease in late onset families. Science 1993;261:921–3

15. Strittmatter WJ, Saunders AM, Schmechel D, et al. Apolipoprotein E: High-avidity binding to beta-amyloid and increased frequency of type 4 allele in late-onset familial Alzheimer disease. Proc Natl Acad Sci (USA) 1993;90:1977–81

16. Blacker D, Haines JL, Rodes L, et al. ApoE-4 and age at onset of Alzheimer's disease: The NIMH genetics initiative. Neurology 1997;48:139–47

17. Premkumar DRD, Cohen DL, Hedera P, et al. Apolipoprotein E-ε4 alleles in cerebral amyloid angiopathy and cerebrovascular pathology associated with Alzheimer's disease. Am J Pathol 1996;148:2083–95

18. Greenberg SM, Briggs ME, Hyman BT, et al. Apolipoprotein E ε4 is associated with the presence and earlier onset of hemorrhage in cerebral amyloid angiopathy. Stroke 1996;27:1333–7

19. Shimano H, Ishibashi S, Murase T. Plasma apolipoproteins in patients with multi-infarct dementia. Atherosclerosis 1989;79:257–60

20. Slooter AJC, Ming-Xin T, van Duijn CM, et al. Apolipoprotein E ε4 and the risk of dementia with stroke. J Am Med Assoc 1997;277:818–21

21. Masters CL, Simms G, Weinman NA, et al. Amyloid plaque core protein in Alzheimer disease and Down syndrome. Proc Natl Acad Sci (USA) 1985;82: 4245–9

22. Wisniewski T, Lalowski M, Golabek AA, et al. Is Alzheimer's disease an apolipoprotein E amyloidosis? Lancet 1995;345:956–8

23. Wisniewski T, Palha JA, Ghiso J, et al. S182 protein in Alzheimer's disease neuritic plaques. Lancet 1995; 346:1366

24. Prelli F, Castaño EM, Glenner GG, et al. Differences between vascular and plaque core amyloid in Alzheimer's disease. J Neurochem 1988;51:648–51

25. Joachim CL, Duffy LK, Morris JH, et al. Protein chemical and immunocytochemical studies of meningovascular beta-amyloid protein in Alzheimer's disease and normal aging. Brain Res 1988; 474:100–11

26. Miller DL, Papayannopoulos IA, Styles J, et al. Peptide compositions of the cerebrovascular and senile plaque core amyloid deposits of Alzheimer's disease. Arch Biochem Biophys 1993;301:41–52

27. Wisniewski T, Lalowski M, Levy E, et al. The amino acid sequence of neuritic plaque amyloid from a familial Alzheimer's disease patient. Ann Neurol 1994;35:245–6

28. Glenner GG, Wong CW. Alzheimer's disease: Initial report of the purification and characterization of a novel cerebrovascular amyloid protein. Biochem Biophys Res Commun 1984;120: 885–90

29. Roher AE, Lowenson JD, Clarke S, et al. β-Amyloid (1–42) is a major component of cerebrovascular amyloid deposits: Implications for the pathology of Alzheimer disease. Proc Natl Acad Sci (USA) 1993;90: 10836–40

30. Haass C, Schlossmacher MG, Hung AY, et al. Amyloid beta-peptide is produced by cultured cells during normal metabolism. Nature 1992;359:322–5

31. Seubert P, Vigo-Pelfrey C, Esch F, et al. Isolation and quantification of soluble Alzheimer's beta-peptide from biological fluids. Nature 1992;359:325–7

32. Shoji M, Golde TE, Ghiso J, *et al.* Production of the Alzheimer amyloid beta protein by normal proteolytic processing. *Science* 1992;258:126–9

33. Busciglio J, Gabuzda DH, Matsudaira P, *et al.* Generation of β-amyloid in the secretory pathway in neuronal and non-neuronal cells. *Proc Natl Acad Sci (USA)* 1993;90:2092–6

34. Vigo-Pelfrey C, Lee D, Keim P, *et al.* Characterization of beta-amyloid peptide from human cerebrospinal fluid. *J Neurochem* 1993; 61:1965–8

35. Kang J, Lemaire HG, Unterbeck A, *et al.* The precursor of Alzheimer's disease amyloid A4 protein resembles a cell-surface receptor. *Nature* 1987;325: 733–6

36. Goldgaber D, Lerman MI, McBride OW, *et al.* Characterization and chromosomal localization of a cDNA encoding brain amyloid of Alzheimer's disease. *Science* 1987;235:877–80

37. Robakis NK, Ramakrishna N, Wolfe G, *et al.* Molecular cloning and characterization of a cDNA encoding the neuritic plaque amyloid peptides. *Proc Natl Acad Sci (USA)* 1987;84:4190–4

38. Tanzi RE, Gusella JF, Watkins PC, *et al.* Amyloid β-protein gene: cDNA, mRNA distribution and genetic linkage near the Alzheimer's locus. *Science* 1987;235:880–4

39. Kitaguchi N, Takahashi Y, Tokushima Y, *et al.* Novel precursor of Alzheimer's disease amyloid protein shows protease inhibitory activity. *Nature* 1988;331:530–2

40. Tanzi RE, McClatchy AI, Lamperti ED, *et al.* Protease inhibitor domain encoded by an amyloid precursor mRNA associated with Alzheimer's disease. *Nature* 1988;331:528–30

41. Golde TE, Estus S, Usiak M, *et al.* Expression of β-amyloid protein precursor mRNAs; recognition of a novel alternatively spliced form and quantitation in Alzheimer's disease using PCR. *Neuron* 1990; 4:253–67

42. Lemaire HG, Salbaum JM, Multhaup G, *et al.* The Pre A4695 precursor protein of Alzheimer's disease A4 amyloid is encoded by 16 exons. *Nucleic Acids Res* 1989;17:517–22

43. Konig G, Monning U, Czech C, *et al.* Identification and differential expression of a novel alternative splice isoform of the β A4 amyloid precursor protein (APP) mRNA in leukocytes and brain microglial cells. *J Biol Chem* 1992;267:10804–9

44. Esch FS, Keim PS, Beattie EC, *et al.* Cleavage of amyloid β peptide during constitutive processing of its precursor. *Science* 1990;248:1122–4

45. van Nostrand WE, Schmaier AH, Farrow JS, *et al.* Protease nexin-II (amyloid β-protein precursor): A platelet alpha granule protein. *Science* 1990;248: 745–8

46. Sisodia SS, Koo EH, Beyreuther K, *et al.* Evidence that β-amyloid protein in Alzheimer's disease is not derived by normal processing. *Science* 1990; 248:492–5

47. Wang R, Meschia JF, Cotter RJ, *et al.* Secretion of the β/A4 amyloid precursor protein. *J Biol Chem* 1991;266:16960–4

48. Wisniewski T, Frangione B. Molecular biology of Alzheimer's amyloid – Dutch variant. *Mol Neurobiol* 1992;6:75–86

49. Wisniewski T, Ghiso J, Frangione B. Peptides homologous to the amyloid protein of Alzheimer's disease containing a glutamine for glutamic acid substitution have accelerated amyloid fibril formation. *Biochem Biophys Res Commun* 1991;179: 1247–54

50. Castaño EM, Prelli F, Wisniewski T, *et al.* Fibrillogenesis in Alzheimer's disease of amyloid beta peptides and apolipoprotein E. *Biochem J* 1995;306: 599–604

51. Clements A, Walsh DM, Williams CH, *et al.* Effects of the mutation Glu^{22} to Gln and Ala^{21} to Gly on the aggregation of a synthetic fragment of the Alzheimer's amyloid β/A4 peptide. *Neurosci Lett* 1993;161:17–20

52. Citron M, Oltersdorf T, Haass C, et al. Mutation of the beta-amyloid precursor protein in familial Alzheimer's disease increases beta-protein production. Nature 992;360:672–4

53. Citron M, Vigo-Pelfrey C, Teplow DB, et al. Excessive production of amyloid β-amyloid precursor protein gene. Proc Natl Acad Sci (USA) 1993;91: 11993–7

54. Suzuki N, Cheung TT, Cai TT, et al. An increased percentage of long amyloid β protein secreted by familial amyloid β protein precursor (βPP717) mutants. Science 1994;264:1336–40

55. Younkin SG. Evidence that Aβ 42 is the real culprit in Alzheimer's disease. Ann Neurol 1995;37:287–8

56. Jarrett JT, Lansbury PT Jr. Seeding "one-dimensional crystallization" of amyloid: A pathogenic mechanism in Alzheimer's disease and scrapie? Cell 1993;73:1055–8

57. Lendon CL, Ashall F, Goate AM. Exploring the etiology of Alzheimer disease using molecular genetics. J Am Med Assoc 1997;277:825–31

58. Kwok JBJ, Taddei K, Hallupp M, et al. Two novel (M233T and R278T) presenilin-1 mutations in early-onset Alzheimer's disease pedigrees and preliminary evidence for association of presenilin-1 mutations with a novel phenotype. Neuroreport 1997;8:1537–42

59. Cruts M, Van Broeckhoven C. Presenilin mutations in Alzheimer's disease. Hum Mutation 1998; 11:183–90

60. Wisniewski T, Dowjat WK, Buxbaum JD, et al. A novel Polish presenilin-1 mutation (P117L) is associated with familial Alzheimer's disease and leads to death as early as the age of 28 years. Neuroreport 1998;9:217–21

61. Wegiel J, Wisniewski HM, Kuchna I, et al. Cell-type specific enhancement of amyloid-β deposition in a novel presenilin-1 mutation (P117L). J Neuropathol Exp Neurol 1998;57:831–8

62. Doan A, Thinakaran G, Borchelt DR, et al. Protein topology of presenilin 1. Neuron 1996;17:1023–30

63. Li X, Greenwald I. Membrane topology of the C. elegans SEL-12 presenilin. Neuron 1996;17:1015–21

64. Lehmann S, Chiesa R, Harris DA. Evidence for a six-transmembrane domain structure of presenilin 1. J Biol Chem 1997;272:12047–51

65. Cribbs DH, Chen LS, Bende SM, et al. Widespread neuronal expression of the presenilin-1 early-onset Alzheimer's disease gene in the murine brain. Am J Pathol 1996;148:1797–1806

66. Kovacs D, Fausett HJ, Page KJ, et al. Alzheimer associated presenilin 1 and 2: Neuronal expression in brain and localization to intracellular membranes in mammalian cells. Nature Med 1996;2:224–9

67. Uchihara T, Hamid HK, Duyckaerts C, et al. Widespread immunoreactivity of presenilin in neurons of normal and Alzheimer's disease brains: Double-labeling immunohistochemical study. Acta Neuropathol 1996;92:325–30

68. Giannakopoulos P, Bouras C, Kovari E, et al. Presenilin-1 immunoreactive neurons are preserved in late-onset Alzheimer's disease. Am J Pathol 1997; 150:429–36

69. Elder GA, Tezapsidis N, Carter J, et al. Identification and neuron specific expression of the S182/presenilin 1 protein in human and rodent brains. J Neurosci Res 1996;45:308–20

70. Weber LL, Leissring MA, Yang AJ, et al. Presenilin-1 immunoreactivity is localized intracellularly in Alzheimer's disease brain, but not detected in amyloid plaques. Exp Neurol 1997;143:37–44

71. Lah JJ, Heilman CJ, Nash NR, et al. Light and electron microscopic localization of presenilin-1 in primate brain. J Neurosci 1997;17:1971–80

72. Thinakaran G, Borchelt DR, Lee M, et al. Endoproteolysis of presenilin 1 and accumulation of processed derivatives in vivo. Neuron 1996;17:181–90

73. Levitan D, Greenwald I. Facilitation of lin-12-mediated signalling by sel-12, a Caenorhabditis elegans S182 Alzheimer's disease gene. Nature 1996;377: 351–4

74. L'Hernault SW, Arduengo PM. Mutation of a putative sperm membrane protein in *Caenorhabditis elegans* prevents sperm differentiation but not its associated meiotic divisions. *J Cell Biol* 1992;119:55–68

75. Wong PC, Zhen H, Chen H, *et al.* Presenilin I is required for Notch I and DIII expression in the paraxial mesoderm. *Nature (London)* 1997; 387:288–92

76. Wisniewski T, Dowjat W, Permanne B, *et al.* Presenilin is associated with Alzheimer's disease amyloid. *Am J Pathol* 1997;151:601–10

77. Levey AI, Heilman CJ, Lah JJ, *et al.* Presenilin-1 protein expression in familial and sporadic Alzheimer's disease. *Ann Neurol* 1997;41:742–53

78. De Strooper B, Saftig P, Craessaerts K, *et al.* Deficiency of presenilin-1 inhibits the normal cleavage of amyloid precursor protein. *Nature* 1998;391:387–90

79. Scheuner D, Eckman C, Jensen M, *et al.* Secreted amyloid β-protein similar to that in the senile plaques of Alzheimer's disease is increased *in vivo* by the presenilin 1 and 2 and APP mutations linked to familial Alzheimer's disease. *Nature Med* 1996;2:864–70

80. Duff K, Eckman C, Zehr C, *et al.* Increased amyloid-β42(43) in brains of mice expressing mutant presenilin 1. *Nature* 1996;383:710–3

81. Citron M, Westaway D, Xia WM, *et al.* Mutant presenilins of Alzheimer's disease increase production of 42-residue amyloid β-protein in both transfected cells and transgenic mice. *Nature Med* 1997; 3:67–72

82. Borchelt DR, Thinakaran G, Eckman CB, *et al.* Familial Alzheimer's disease-linked presenilin I variants elevate Aβ1–42/1–40 ratio *in vitro* and *in vivo*. *Neuron* 1996;17:1005–13

83. Lemere CA, Lopera F, Kosik KS, *et al.* The E280A presenilin I Alzheimer mutation produced Aβ42 deposition and severe cerebellar pathology. *Nature Med* 1996;2:1146–50

84. Borchelt DR, Ratovitski T, Van Lare J, *et al.* Accelerated amyloid deposition in the brains of transgenic mice coexpressing mutant presenilin I and amyloid precursor proteins. *Neuron* 1997;19: 939–45

85. Holcomb L, Gordon MN, McGowan E, *et al.* Accelerated Alzheimer-type phenotype in transgenic mice carrying both mutant amyloid precursor protein and presenilin I transgenes. *Nat Genet* 1998;4:97–100

86. Vito P, Lacana E, D'Adamio L. Interfering with apoptosis: Ca^{2+}-binding protein ALG-2 and Alzheimer's disease gene *ALG-3*. *Science* 1996; 271:521–5

87. Wolozin B, Iwasaki K, Vito P, *et al.* Participation of presenilin 2 in apoptosis: Enhanced basal activity conferred by an Alzheimer mutation. *Science* 1996;274:1710–3

88. Guo Q, Sopher BL, Furukawa K, *et al.* Alzheimer's presenilin mutation sensitizes neural cells to apoptosis induced by trophic factor withdrawal and amyloid β-peptide: Involvement of calcium and oxyradicals. *J Neurosci* 1997;17:4212–22

89. Wolozin B, Alexander P, Palacino J. Regulation of apoptosis by presenilin I. *Neurobiol Aging* 1998;19: S23–7

90. Bouras C, Giannakopoulos P, Schioi J, *et al.* Presenilin-1 polymorphism and Alzheimer's disease. *Lancet* 1996;347:1185–6

91. Podlisny MB, Citron M, Amarante P, *et al.* Presenilin proteins undergo heterogeneous endoproteolysis between Thr_{291} and Ala_{299} and occur as stable N- and C-terminal fragments in normal and Alzheimer brain tissue. *Neurobiol Dis* 1997;3:325–37

92. Namba Y, Tomonaga M, Kawasaki H, *et al.* Apolipoprotein E immunoreactivity in cerebral amyloid deposits and neurofibrillary tangles in Alzheimer's disease and kuru plaque amyloid in Creutzfeldt– Jakob disease. *Brain Res* 1991;541:163–6

93. Wisniewski T, Frangione B. Apolipoprotein E: A pathological chaperone protein in patients with cerebral and systemic amyloid. *Neurosci Lett* 1992; 135:235–8

94. Beissinger M, Buchner J. How chaperones fold proteins. *Biol Chem* 1998;379:245–59

95. Mahley RW. Apolipoprotein E: Cholesterol transport protein with expanding role in cell biology. *Science* 1988;240:622–30

96. Schmechel DE, Saunders AM, Strittmatter WJ, et al. Increased amyloid beta-peptide deposition in cerebral cortex as a consequence of apolipoprotein E genotype in late-onset Alzheimer disease. *Proc Natl Acad Sci (USA)* 1993;90:9649–53

97. Rebeck GW, Reiter JS, Strickland DK, et al. Apolipoprotein E in sporadic Alzheimer's disease: Allelic variation and receptor interactions. *Neuron* 1993;11: 575–80

98. Golabek AA, Soto C, Vogel T, et al. The interaction between apolipoprotein E and Alzheimer's amyloid β-peptide is dependent on β-peptide conformation. *J Biol Chem* 1996;271:10602–6

99. Naslund J, Thyberg J, Tjernberg LO, et al. Characterization of stable complexes involving apolipoprotein E and the amyloid beta peptide in Alzheimer's disease brain. *Neuron* 1995;15:219–28

100. Wisniewski T, Castaño EM, Golabek AA, et al. Acceleration of Alzheimer's fibril formation by apolipoprotein E *in vitro*. *Am J Pathol* 1994;145: 1030–5

101. Ma J, Yee A, Brewer HB Jr., et al. Amyloid-associated proteins alpha 1-antichymotrypsin and apolipoprotein E promote assembly of Alzheimer beta-protein into filaments. *Nature* 1994;372:92–4

102. Sanan DA, Weisgraber KH, Russell SJ, et al. Apolipoprotein E associates with beta amyloid peptide of Alzheimer's disease to form novel monofibrils. Isoform apoE4 associates more efficiently than apoE3. *J Clin Invest* 1994;94:860–9

103. Bales KR, Verina T, Dodel RC, et al. Lack of apolipoprotein E dramatically reduces amyloid β-peptide deposition. *Nature Gen* 1997;17:263–4

104. Ghersi-Egea JF, Gorevic PD, Ghiso J, et al. Fate of cerebrospinal fluid-borne amyloid β-peptide: Rapid clearance into blood and appreciable accumulation by cerebral arteries. *J Neurochem* 1996; 67:880–3

105. Permanne B, Perez C, Soto C, et al. Detection of apolipoprotein E dimeric soluble amyloid β complexes in Alzheimer's disease brain supernatants. *Biochem Biophys Res Commun* 1997;240:715–20

106. Holtzman DM, Bales KR, Wu S, et al. Expression of human apolipoprotein E reduces amyloid β deposition in a mouse model of Alzheimer's disease. *J Clin Invest* 1999;103:15–21

107. Linton MF, Gish R, Hubl ST, et al. Phenotypes of apoB and apoE after liver transplantation. *J Clin Invest* 1991;88:270–81

108. Hardy J. New insights into the genetics of Alzheimer's disease. *Ann Med* 1996;28:255–8

109. Yamaguchi H, Hirai S, Morimatsu M, et al. Diffuse type of senile plaques in the brains of Alzheimer-type dementia. *Acta Neuropathol* 1988;77:113–9

110. Tagliavini F, Giaccone G, Frangione B, et al. Preamyloid deposits in the cerebral cortex of patients with Alzheimer's disease and nondemented individuals. *Neurosci Lett* 1988;93:191–6

111. Wisniewski HM, Bancher C, Barcikowska M, et al. Spectrum of morphological appearance of amyloid deposits in AD. *Acta Neuropathol* 1989;78:337–47

112. Yamazaki T, Yamaguchi H, Okamoto K, et al. Ultrastrutural localization of argyrophilic substances in diffuse plaques of Alzheimer-type dementia demonstrated by methenamine silver staining. *Acta Neuropathol* 1991;81:540–5

113. Yamaguchi H, Nakazato Y, Shoji M, et al. Ultrastructure of diffuse plaques in senile dementia of the Alzheimer type: Comparison with primitive plaques. *Acta Neuropathol* 1991;82:13–20

114. Crystal HA, Dickson DW, Sliwinski MJ, et al. Pathological markers associated with normal aging and dementia in the elderly. *Ann Neurol* 1993;34: 566–73

115. Davies P, Duyckaerts C, Beyreuther K, et al. A4 amyloid protein deposition and the diagnosis of Alzheimer's disease: Prevalence in aged brains determined by immunohistochemistry compared with conventional neuropathological techniques. *Neurology* 1988;38:1688–93

116. Delaere P, Duyckaerts C, Beyreuther K, et al. Large amounts of neocortical βA4 deposits without neuritc plaques or tangles in a psychometrically assessed nondemented case. *Neurosci Lett* 1990; 116:87–93

117. Wisniewski HM, Wegiel J, Popovitch ER. Age-associated development of diffuse and thioflavine-S-positive plaques in Down syndrome. *Dev Brain Dysfunct* 1994;7:330–9

118. Kida E, Choi-Miura NH, Wisniewski KE. Deposition of apolipoproteins E and J in senile plaques is topographically determined in both Alzheimer's disease and Down's syndrome brain. *Brain Res* 1995;685:211–6

119. Lemere CA, Blusztajn JK, Yamaguchi H, et al. Sequence of deposition of heterogeneous amyloid β-peptides and APO E in Down syndrome: Implications for initial events in amyloid plaque formation. *Neurobiol Dis* 1996;3:16–32

120. Polvikoski T, Sulkava R, Haltia M, et al. Apolipoprotein E, dementia, and cortical deposition of β-amyloid protein. *N Eng J Med* 1995;333:1242–7

121. Kosik KS, Coleman P. Is β-amyloid neurotoxic? *Neurobiol Aging* 1992;13:535–627

122. Pike CJ, Burdick D, Walencewicz AJ, et al. Neurodegeneration induced by beta-amyloid peptides *in vitro*: The role of peptide assembly state. *J Neurosci* 1993;13:1676–87

123. Simmons LK, May PC, Tomaselli KJ, et al. Secondary structure of amyloid beta peptide correlates with neurotoxic activity *in vitro*. *Mol Pharmacol* 1994;45:373–9

124. Ueda K, Fukui Y, Kageyama H. Amyloid beta protein induces neuronal cell death: Neurotoxic properties of aggregated amyloid beta protein. *Brain Res* 1994;639:240–4

125. Lorenzo A, Yankner BA. Beta-amyloid neurotoxicity requires fibril formation and is inhibited by congo red. *Proc Natl Acad Sci (USA)* 1994;91: 12243–7

126. Games D, Adams D, Alessandrini R, et al. Alzheimer-type neuropathology in transgenic mice overexpressing V717F β-amyloid precursor protein. *Nature* 1995;373:523–7

127. Hsiao KK, Chapman P, Nilsen S, et al. Correlative memory deficits, Aβ elevation and amyloid plaques in transgenic mice. *Science* 1996;274:99–102

128. Irizarry MC, Soriano F, McNamara M, et al. Aβ deposition is associated with neuropil changes, but not with overt neuronal loss in the human amyloid precursor protein V717F (PDAPP) transgenic mouse. *J Neurosci* 1997;17:7053–9

129. Irizarry MC, McNamara M, Fedorchak K, et al. APP$_{Sw}$ transgenic mice develop age-related Aβ deposits and neuropil abnormalities, but no neuronal loss in CA1. *J Neuropath Exp Neurol* 1997; 56:965–973

130. Calhoun ME, Wiederhold KH, Abramowski D, et al. Neuron loss in APP transgenic mice. *Nature* 1998;396:755–6

131. Johnson-Wood K, Lee M, Motter R, et al. Amyloid precursor protein processing and Aβ42 deposition in a transgenic mouse model of Alzheimer's disease. *Proc Natl Acad Sci (USA)* 1997;94:1550–5

132. Wisniewski T, Lalowski M, Bobik M, et al. Amyloid β 1–42 deposits do not lead to Alzheimer's neuritic plaques in aged dogs. *Biochem J* 1996;313:575–80

133. Lalowski M, Golabek AA, Lemere CA, et al. The "non-amyloidogenic" p3 fragment (Aβ17–42) is a major constituent of Down syndrome cerebellar preamyloid. *J Biol Chem* 1996;271:33623–31

134. Hutton M, Lendon CL, Rizzu P, et al. Association of missense and 5'-splice-site mutations in tau and the inherited dementia FTDP-17. *Nature* 1998;393: 702–5

135. Vogel G. Tau protein mutations confirmed as neuron killers. *Science* 1998;280:1524–5

9 Genetics of Alzheimer's disease

Judes Poirier, Doris Dea and Marc Danik

Introduction

Alzheimer's disease (AD) is considered today to be a multifactorial disease with a strong genetic component. It is generally agreed that the disease can be subdivided into two distinct categories: the (so-called) familial and the sporadic forms of the disease. The discovery of genetic linkage and the identification of genes responsible for diseases such as AD has revolutionized our understanding of this disorder, which was believed to have an obscure and complex etiology. The identification of specific mutations in genes that are known to be linked to AD has changed how we perceive the nature of the molecular changes responsible for the pathophysiological process that characterizes AD. The familial form of AD accounts for roughly 15% of all cases worldwide, whereas the (so-called) sporadic form of AD represents 85% of the remaining cases and is generally believed to be of late onset, occurring after 65 years of age.

Family history

A family history of AD is one of the most consistent risk factors, increasing disease risk by approximately fourfold at any age. Statistical corrections for cases 'censored' as a result of death from other causes have suggested that as many as 75% of cases of AD may be familial. The familial disease occurs in a pattern consistent with autosomal-dominant inheritance, affecting 50% of subjects who achieve the age of risk.

Familial clustering, however, need not be genetic in origin. Studies in twins have shown that concordance of AD (40–42%) is similar in both 'identical' and non-identical twins. Even in concordant twins, the time of disease onset may vary by a decade or more, thereby implying environmental factors. Although the number of twin pairs studied has been small, these data raise doubt that the common forms of AD are essentially genetic in origin.

At present, the conservative position is that genetics plays a variable role in the causation of AD. In some families, a genetic abnormality plays a dominant role, leading to the development of the disease in virtually any affected individual who reaches the age of risk. In other families, a genetic aberration may predispose members to develop the disease, but its clinical expression may depend on environmental factors. In some individuals with sporadic AD, genetics may not be an important contributing factor. However, the recent discovery that the apolipoprotein E4 (apo E4) allele is a marker for both familial and sporadic late-onset AD raises the possibility of a role for genetics in sporadic subjects.

Familial Alzheimer's disease

Molecular genetic studies have identified several different genetic loci believed to be linked to the presence of AD in the general population. The known genetic causes of AD, which include mutations of the amyloid precursor protein (APP) gene and of the two presenilin genes, account for around

5% of all AD cases worldwide. These rare mutations are transmitted as autosomal-dominant traits in certain families in Europe, North America and Asia. Although much has been learned from studies of these gene mutations, the molecular mechanism(s) underlying the sporadic form of AD is much more complex and requires a different approach. Indeed, the chromosomal locus referred to as apo E4 has been linked to both the late-onset familial form as well as the sporadic form of AD. The majority of patients considered to be sporadic cases probably arise as the result of several genetic anomalies, each making an independent contribution to the overall phenotype and pathophysiological process. It is suspected that at least one, and most probably several, additional mutations remain to be identified as only 50% of all AD cases have been associated with specific genetic anomalies.

Apolipoprotein E4 and Alzheimer's disease

Apolipoproteins are protein components of lipoprotein particles. The latter are macromolecular complexes that carry lipids such as cholesterol and phospholipids from one cell to another within a tissue or between organs. Some apolipoproteins regulate extracellular enzymatic reactions related to lipid homeostasis whereas others are ligands for cell surface receptors that mediate lipoprotein uptake into cells and their subsequent metabolism.

Apo E is a component of several classes of plasma and cerebrospinal fluid lipoproteins. The putative three-dimensional structure of purified human apo E is shown in Figure 1. In humans, after the liver, the brain is the most important site of apo E expression.

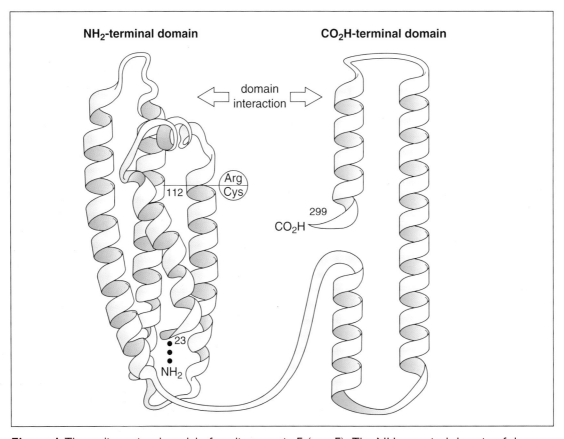

Figure 1 Three-dimensional model of apolipoprotein E (apo E). The NH_2-terminal domain of the protein contains the receptor-binding region of apo E (residues 136–150) whereas the CO_2H-terminal domain contains the major lipoprotein-binding determinants of apo E. Positions 112 and 158 distinguish apo E3, apo E4 and apo E2. Arg, arginine; Cys, cysteine. Modified from reference 3

Apo E has been shown to be synthesized and secreted by glial cells, predominantly astrocytes, but not by neurons. However, the latter may have apo E immunoreactivity *in vivo* due to their capability to bind and internalize apo E, as demonstrated by hippocampal neuronal cell cultures (Figure 2). Several cell surface receptors for apo E are known to be expressed on one or many of the different cell types that constitute the brain parenchyma. These receptors are members of a single family and include the low-density lipoprotein (LDL) receptor, the very low-density (VLDL) receptor, the apo E2 receptor (apo-ER2), the LDL receptor-related protein (LRP) and the megalin / gp330 receptor.

The importance of apo E in lipid homeostasis in the brain is underscored by the fact that major plasma apolipoproteins such as apo B and apo A-I are not synthesized in the central nervous system (CNS). Early data from animal lesion paradigms, such as sciatic nerve crush and entorhinal cortex lesions, suggested that apo E plays a role in the coordinated storage and redistribution of cholesterol and phospholipids among cells within the remodeling area.

Apo E is now believed to have an important role not only in reactive synaptogenesis by delivering lipids to remodeling and sprouting neurons in response to tissue injury, but also in physiological ongoing synaptic plasticity and maintenance of neuronal integrity as well as in cholinergic activity.

Three alleles (ϵ2, ϵ3 and ϵ4) at a single gene locus on the long arm of chromosome 19 code for the common isoforms of apo E, namely, apo E2, apo E3 and apo E4. This allelic heterogeneity gives rise to a protein polymorphism at two positions: residue 112 and residue 158 on the mature protein. The presence of either a cysteine or an arginine at these polymorphic sites leads to a charge difference detectable by isoelectric focusing. The most common apo E allele is ϵ3, which has a frequency >60% in all populations. Allelic distribution in a typical elderly white population is approximately 8% for ϵ2, 78% for ϵ3 and 14% for ϵ4. The relative allelic frequencies in other ethnic groups such as black Americans, Hispanics and Japanese were reported to be similar among elderly populations.

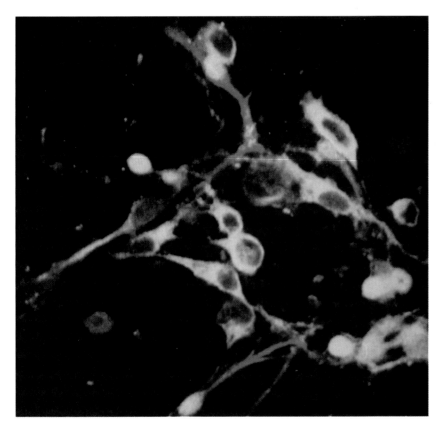

Figure 2 Low-power ($\times$25) laser confocal micrograph of human apo E4 immunoreactivity in primary neuronal cells from rats exposed to reconstituted human apo E4 for 3 min. Apo E immunoreactivity is predominantly localized in neuronal cells (green) whereas glial fibrillary acidic protein (GFAP) immunoreactivity identifies the contaminating primary astrocytes (orange)

Recently, the apo E ε4 allele was found to be over-represented in groups of both familial and sporadic cases of late-onset AD (LOAD), which accounts for approximately 90% of all AD cases. The ε4 allele frequency was shown to be significantly higher (around threefold, or 40–50%) in the AD population. Interestingly, a sharp decline in the prevalence of the ε4 allele was observed in very old subjects (>85 years), suggesting the presence of a very late-onset form of AD and consistent with the increased risk of coronary heart disease in those with apo E ε4.

The emergence of apo E4 as a major risk factor for AD has since been confirmed in more than 100 studies worldwide. Estimates indicate that more than half of the susceptibility to AD is associated with the apo E locus. Inheritance of one or two apo E ε4 alleles is associated with a 'dose'-related higher risk and younger age of onset distribution of AD. Individuals with one apo E ε4 allele have a two- to fourfold increased risk of developing LOAD compared with those without the apo E ε4 allele whereas subjects who are homozygous for ε4 have a five- to 34-fold increased risk. The apo E ε4–AD association is strongest in Japanese subjects, followed by whites, and is apparently weaker among black Americans and Hispanics. The effect of the least common ε2 allele appears to consist of decreasing the risk and increasing the age of onset compared with the common ε3 allele; therefore, the ε2 allele is considered to be protective. Indeed, the ε2 allele is slightly underrepresented among AD patients, although there are reports to the contrary in some populations. Meta-analysis of 40 studies representing nearly 30 000 apo E alleles concluded that the ε4 allele represents a major risk factor for AD in all ethnic groups and across all ages in the range 40–90 years, but that the effect diminishes after age 70 years.

Increasing the dose of ε4 allele is also associated with an earlier age of onset of AD. In families with LOAD, the mean age of onset was reported to decrease from 84 to 68 years as the number of ε4 alleles increased from 0 to 2. Likewise, a decrease in the average age of onset (from 78 to 70 years) as a function of the ε4 allele copy number was found in sporadic cases with LOAD. The use of homogene-ous populations of subjects in terms of age of onset, severity and duration of the disease allowed disease progression to be monitored while reducing intrinsic variability due to non-linear decline in function in AD patients. When such populations enrolled in clinical drug trials (patient mean age of 75 years) were analyzed, the placebo arm revealed a clear difference in the rate of progression, as determined by variation in the Alzheimer's Disease Assessment Scale-Cognition (ADAS-Cog) over a 6-month period. The non-ε4 mild-to-moderate subgroup showed a significantly faster rate of progression compared with the ε4 subgroup.

In addition to the effects of increasing risk and lowering age of onset, increasing the number of ε4 alleles is also known to correlate with augmentation of the number of senile plaques and neurofibrillary tangles (NFTs) in the brain of sporadic late-onset subjects, although the latter association is more controversial and could be attributed to the correlation between NFTs and duration of illness associated with apo E ε4 carriers. Immunochemical localization of apo E in extracellular amyloid deposits, including vascular deposits, and in neurons containing NFTs, suggested that apo E was involved in AD.

These results led to the study of the interactions of apo E3 and apo E4 with the main constituent of senile plaque deposits, the amyloid β-peptide, and with microtubule-associated protein tau. These studies revealed isoform-specific differences in the *in vitro* affinity of apo E for amyloid and for tau. However, discrepancies among the results obtained from these studies make it difficult to explain the correlations between the ε4 copy number and the histopathological marker's density. Although the importance of apo E in triggering amyloid β-peptide deposition in the brain of amyloid precursor protein transgenic mice has recently been demonstrated, the pathogenicity of the protein interaction as the primary cause or the consequence of dying neurons is still under debate.

Brain levels of cholesterol and choline, a precursor of the neurotransmitter acetylcholine, were shown to be reduced in AD patients. Moreover, losses of cholinergic neurons and / or choline acetyltransferase (ChAT) activities are other well-known features of AD. It is interesting to note that the apo E ε4 allele copy number is inversely related to residual brain ChAT activity and nicotinic receptor binding sites in both the hippocampal formation and the temporal cortex of AD patients. Furthermore, the density of cholinergic neurons in the basal forebrain, which represents the primary cholinergic input to these areas, was significantly reduced in ε4 allele carriers compared with non-ε4 AD patients or control subjects. Increased cholinergic neuron vulnerability and reduced plasticity in ε4 carriers supports the hypothesis of a less efficient delivery of cholesterol and phospholipids (including donor intermediates of choline) to cells of the CNS as a consequence of lower apo E expression in these subjects.

Recently, the role of apo E polymorphisms as potent pharmacogenetic markers was validated by several independent groups, which have shown that the presence or absence of ε4 alleles (in combination with gender) in a given subject markedly affects the response to several antidementia drugs, including tacrine, metrifonate, S12024 and, more recently, selegiline.

The emerging field of AD pharmacogenetics will probably have a significant impact on the development of the next generation of antidementia drugs. Subjects participating in drug trials will be required to undergo genetic testing to assess the pharmacogenetic contribution of each of the apo E alleles on both the efficacy and toxicity of the new medication. More important, the contribution of novel risk factors, such as the presenilins, butyrylcholinesterase K, α₁-antichymotrypsin and LDL receptor-related proteins, to the pathophysiology of AD will become an integral part of the genetic profiling process of patients. In effect, AD may be among the first, if not THE first, to be treated in the context of molecular medicine where genetic information is combined with rigorous clinical assessment to select 'the best drug for the right patient'.

Amyloid precursor protein

The first gene to be identified in association with familial AD was the amyloid precursor protein (APP) gene (Figure 3). The APP gene encodes for a transcript which, once translated, encodes for a single transmembrane-spanning polypeptide of roughly 750 amino acids. Alternative splicing of

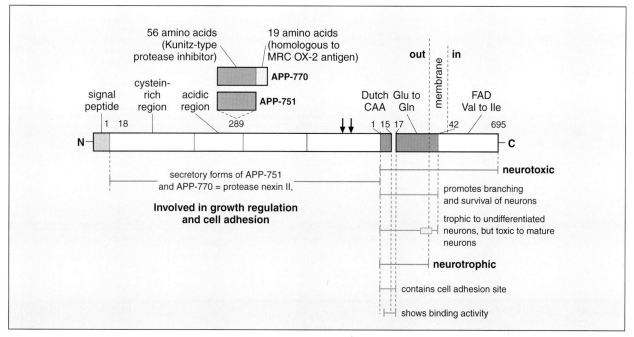

Figure 3 Human amyloid precursor protein, including its metabolites and fragments, and their putative functions and properties

exon7and exon 8 results in a polypeptide of 695 amino acids, which is expressed at very high concentrations in the CNS. The so-called APP precursor protein is known to undergo a series of proteolytic cleavages resulting in the production of a small, 40–42 amino acid peptide referred to as the Aβ-peptide.

The precise function of APP is currently unknown, but recent evidence suggests a preeminent role in the maintenance of cholesterol homeostasis, and an indirect involvement during reinnervation and synaptic replacement. Onset at around the age of 50 years is characteristic of familial AD pedigrees associated with mutation of the APP gene; at least eight mutations, at positions 665, 670, 673, 692, 693, 713, 716 and 717, have been identified as causative of early-to-late-onset familial AD (Table 1). The clinical features of affected subjects include prominent early myoclonus and seizures, depression and lack of insight into their cognitive deficit. Naming skills, on the other hand, are relatively well preserved. Magnetic resonance imaging (MRI) performed on these families reveal early hippocampal atrophy. Patients' mean age of onset varies from in the early 40s to the mid-50s.

The mechanism(s) by which selected APP mutations cause AD remains unclear at present. The most obvious explanation is that the mutations of the APP gene cause an overproduction of the so-called neurotoxic form of β-amyloid, referred to as the 1–42 / 1–43 β-peptides. Polymerization of these fibers could then lead to the development of senile plaque in the brain of AD patients, with a concomitant impact on cerebral integrity. The primary issue that needs to be clarified regarding the so-called amyloid cascade hypothesis is whether amyloid plaque deposition is a primary event in the cascade that leads to cell death in the brain of AD patients or, alternatively, whether the intracellular production of these toxic peptides directly affects neuronal survival as well as fibrilization and amyloid deposition. Recent evidence obtained from transgenic animal models of amyloid deposition tends to support the latter hypothesis, with amyloid deposition playing a secondary role with little or no impact on neuronal survival.

Presenilin 1

Following the discovery that only a portion of the familial cases of AD is explained by the presence of a mutation in the APP gene, several independent investigators undertook the search for other candidate genes that could be involved in the remaining familial forms of the disease. These studies identified a series of polymorphic genetic markers located

Table 1 Missense mutations of the β-amyloid precursor protein gene

Codon	Mutation	Phenotype
665	Gln → Asp	Late-onset AD; no segregation
670/671	Lys–Met → Asn–Leu	Familial AD; increased β-amyloid production
692	Ala → Gly	Familial AD plus cerebral hemorrhage; increased β-amyloid production
693	Glu → Gly	Late-onset AD; no segregation
	Glu → Gln	HCHWA-D
713	Ala → Val	Schizophrenia; no segregation
	Ala → Thr	AD; no segregation
717	Val → Ile	Familial AD; increased long β-amyloid isoforms
	Val → Phe	Familial AD
	Val → Gly	Familial AD

HCHWA-D, hereditary cerebral hemorrhage with amyloidosis, Dutch type; modified from reference 5

on chromosomes 14 and 19. Subsequent genetic analysis narrowed the area of interest to a small locus on chromosome 14. The presenilin 1 (PS1) gene was then isolated using positional cloning strategy, and more than 30 different mutations were found by these independent researchers to cause disease.

The PS1 gene is transcribed in a number of organs and cell types. It appears to be expressed in different neuronal cell types in the hippocampus and cerebellum as well as in the olfactory bulb and striatal areas. According to its putative protein structure in the membrane (Figure 4), there is a concentration of mutations located near or in the highly conserved transmembranous domain of PS1. As yet, no deletions, nonsense mutations or genomic rearrangements have been found in the common form of AD. The biochemical consequences of PS1

mutations are currently being explored, but the function of this particular gene has still not been elucidated.

Mutations in the PS1 gene are associated with family pedigrees in which the age of disease onset is in the late 30s / early 40s. The currently known mutations are listed in Table 2. Patients who have this aggressive form of AD are characterized by early myoclonus and severe seizures which tend to increase with disease severity. Scanning reveals a biparietal bitemporal hypometabolism that is relatively characteristic of affected persons, but there is an additional asymmetrical frontal hypo-metabolism that is particularly marked in the left hemisphere in those with this particular form of AD.

As with mutations of the APP gene, mutations of the PS1 genes are associated with an overproduc-

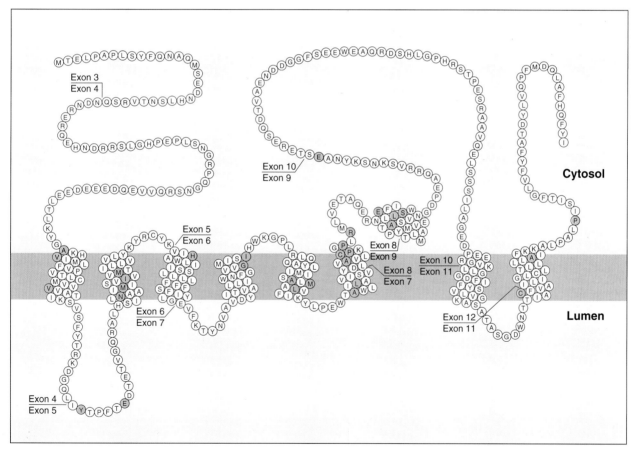

Figure 4 The likely structure of presenilin 1, including exon boundaries. Identified sites of mutations are colored orange. Modified from reference 4

Table 2 Missense mutations of the presenilin 1 and presenilin 2 genes

Codon	Mutation	Phenotype
Presenilin 1		
82	Val → Leu	Familial AD; onset at age 55 years
96	Val → Phe	Familial AD
115	Tyr → His	Familial AD; onset at age 37 years
139	Met → Thr	Familial AD; onset at age 49 years
	Met → Val	Familial AD; onset at age 40 years
143	Ile → Thr	Familial AD; onset at age 35 years
146	Met → Leu	Familial AD; onset at age 45 years
	Met → Val	Familial AD; onset at age 38 years
	Met → Ile	Familial AD; onset at age 40 years
163	His → Arg	Familial AD; onset at age 50 years
	His → Tyr	Familial AD; onset at age 47 years
171	Leu → Pro	Familial AD; onset at age 40 years
209	Gly → Val	Familial AD
213	Ile → Thr	Familial AD
231	Ala → Thr	Familial AD; onset at age 52 years
233	Met → Thr	Familial AD; onset at age 35 years
235	Leu → Pro	Familial AD; onset at age 32 years
246	Ala → Glu	Familial AD; onset at age 55 years
260	Ala → Val	Familial AD; onset at age 40 years
263	Cys → Arg	Familial AD; onset at age 47 years
264	Pro → Leu	Familial AD; onset at age 45 years
267	Pro → Ser	Familial AD; onset at age 35 years
280	Glu → Ala	Familial AD; onset at age 47 years
	Glu → Gly	Familial AD; onset at age 42 years
285	Ala → Val	Familial AD; onset at age 50 years
286	Leu → Val	Familial AD; onset at age 50 years
384	Gly → Ala	Familial AD; onset at age 35 years
392	Leu → Val	Familial AD; onset at age 25–40 years
410	Cys → Tyr	Familial AD; onset at age 48 years
Presenilin 2		
141	Asn → Ile	Familial AD; onset at age 50–65 years
239	Met → Val	Familial AD; onset at age 45–84 years

Modified from reference 5

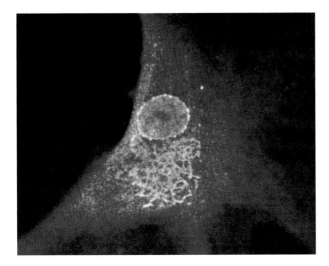

Figure 5 Low-power (×53) laser confocal micrograph of human native fibroblast stained with presenilin 1 antibody (Ab 14) shows immunoreactivity predominantly in the endoplasmic reticulum, perinuclear envelope and Golgi apparatus. From reference 5, with permission

tion of the amyloid β-peptide (1–42)[1] in the brain and fibroblasts of affected subjects. It has been shown that the PS1 protein is localized primarily to the intracellular membrane of the endoplasmic reticulum / Golgi apparatus (Figure 5). Whether or not the increase in β-amyloid is a primary event or secondary to abnormal metabolism of the mutated forms of PS1 remains to be clarified.

Presenilin 2

Following cloning of the PS1 gene on chromosome 14, a similar sequence was identified and subsequently localized on chromosome 1. This polypeptide, referred to as presenilin 2 (PS2), has an open reading frame of around 448 amino acids, with an amino-acid sequence substantially similar to that of PS1 protein, as can be seen in the putative protein structure of PS2 in the membrane (Figure 6).

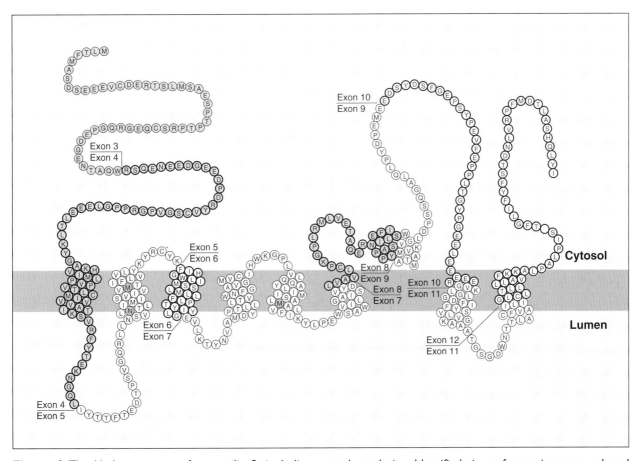

Figure 6 The likely structure of presenilin 2, including exon boundaries. Identified sites of mutations are colored orange. Modified from reference 4

PS2 appears to be more ubiquitously expressed, but less abundant, than PS1. Clues to the function of these presenilins in mammalian cells may be derived from the observation that both PS1 and PS2 share significant amino-acid homology with the *Caenorhabditis elegans* proteins SEL-12 and SPE-4[2]. SEL-12 plays a role in receptor trafficking, localization and recycling of the so-called lin-12, and SPE-4 is involved in cytoplasmic partitioning of proteins. It is, thus, tempting to postulate that the presenilins may be involved in the intracellular trafficking and / or transport of specific proteins inside the cells.

Mutation analysis in familial cases of AD has uncovered two different missense mutations in the PS2 gene in families segregated for early-onset AD (see Table 2 and Figure 6). The first mutation was identified in certain subjects who had the Volga German familial form of AD. The second mutation was discovered in an Italian pedigree. Surprisingly, the range of age of onset in carriers of the PS2 mutation is 40–85 years.

Whether PS1 and PS2 work in concert in the brain remains to be established; however, it should be noted that the pattern of expression of PS1 differs slightly from that of PS2 in the CNS. No more than a few dozens of patients are affected by this particularly rare form of familial AD. Clearly, the relevance of this particular genetic anomaly to a general understanding of AD remains to be established.

Other putative genetic risk factors

Polygenic interactions are now believed to play an important role in the pathophysiology of AD. The most common example of such an interaction is the identification of susceptibility loci in different portions of the human genome. The list of these (so-called) genetic susceptibility factors grows longer every day. To follow is a brief description of the most common genetic risk markers discovered so far and their postulated role in AD.

Low-density lipoprotein receptor-related protein (LRP)

The LDL receptor-related protein (LRP) represents one of the most important apo E receptors expressed by mammalian cells. This multifunctional receptor binds and internalizes lipoprotein complexes containing apo E and apparently may regulate APP metabolism in the brain cell. A common polymorphism in exon 3 has been linked to late-onset sporadic AD, but appears to represent only a small proportion of AD cases worldwide.

Presenilin polymorphism

An intronic presenilin polymorphism was described a few years ago in sporadic AD which shows a strong allelic association in approximately 25% of AD patients. This finding has been independently reproduced in the USA, but not in European countries. The presence of this polymorphism in AD patients does not appear to affect the age of onset, rate of progression or overall pathology.

Butyrylcholinesterase K

A common polymorphism in the butyrylcholinesterase gene called the Kallow (K) allele was reported to be closely associated with a subgroup of sporadic AD patients in a European study. The enzyme is believed to be involved in the regulation of lipid homeostasis in the brain and in the periphery, to catabolize byproducts of drug metabolism and to contribute to the overall metabolism of certain neurotransmitters in the CNS. Whereas two independent studies in Europe and Canada reproduced the original study findings, at least six other separate studies in Europe, Japan, the USA and Australia failed to do so. The presence of this polymorphism does not appear to affect the disease onset, progression or neuropathological features of these patients with sporadic AD.

α_1-Antichymotrypsin

Similarly, a common polymorphism in the α_1-antichymotrypsin gene has also been linked to sporadic AD in a small population sample in the American

GENETICS OF ALZHEIMER'S DISEASE

Midwest. α_1-Antichymotrypsin is an endogenously produced protease inhibitor secreted in the brain as well as peripheral organs. The association between the abnormal allele and sporadic AD has not been reproduced by independent research teams in Boston, Massachusetts and in Florida. European and Japanese AD populations also fail to show an association with these particular polymorphisms.

HLA-DR

Recently, the frequency distribution of certain HLA-DR antigen types has been reported to differ significantly between patients with late-onset AD and age-matched controls. However, a closer look at the results reveals that this is true only for AD patients who carry the apo E4 allele. More recently, it was shown that the presence of the HLA-A2 allele correlates strongly with an earlier age of AD onset. Thus, it is possible that the HLA association may account for the inverse association reported between rheumatoid arthritis and AD. Rheumatoid arthritis is associated with frequencies of 60–70% for the DR4 allele. In these cases, the genetic association appears to have an indirect impact on the pathophysiology of the disease and may serve as a therapeutic target in the treatment of AD.

Chromosome 12 markers

Several independent research teams have identified allelic markers at different positions on chromo-some 12, which appears to segregate with the disease in the familial late-onset form of AD. Some teams report that the susceptibility locus is the LRP gene on chromosome 12 whereas others propose the α-macroglobulin gene; however, a third site is currently emerging by consensus between the loci of these two genes.

Conclusions

The discovery of specific mutations of the APP, PS1 and PS2 genes that co-segregate with the disease in the early-onset forms of AD has allowed important advances to be made in the understanding of the etiology of AD. However, it is the identification of common risk factors, such as the presence of apo E4 in sporadic AD, that has provided the therapeutic targets that may change the lives of the millions of people who suffer from this terrible disease. The extent to which both genetic and non-genetic variables contribute to the central pathological changes of AD needs to be further characterized, using material from living subjects as well as brain samples from pathologically confirmed patients. These data could then serve as a basis for a solid therapeutic strategy aimed at stopping, or even preventing, AD.

References

1. Scheuner D, Eckman C, Jensen M, et al. Secreted amyloid beta-protein similar to that in the senile plaques of Alzheimer's disease is increased in vivo by the presenilin 1 and 2 and APP mutations linked to familial Alzheimer's disease. Nature Med 1996;2:864–70

2. Levitan D, Greenwald I. Facilitation of Lin-12-mediated signalling by Sel-12, a Caenorhabditis elegans S182 Alzheimer's disease gene. Nature (London) 1995;377:351–4

3. Weisgraber KH, Dong LM. Role of apolipoprotein E in Alzheimer's disease: clues from its structure. In Roses AD, Weisgraber KH, Christen Y, eds. Apolipoprotein E and Alzheimer's Disease. Berlin: Springer-Verlag, 1996:11–19

4. Hutton M, Hardy J. The presenilins and Alzheimer's disease. Hum Mol Genet 1997;6:1639–46

5. Fraser PE, Yu G, Levesque G, et al. Molecular genetics of the presenilins in Alzheimer's disease. In Younkin SG, Tanzi RE, Christen Y, eds. Presenilins and Alzheimer's Disease. Berlin: Springer-Verlag, 1998:1–10

Selected bibliography

Apolipoprotein E

Arendt T, Schindler C, Bruckner MK, et al. Plastic neuronal remodeling is impaired in patients with Alzheimer's disease carrying apolipoprotein ∊4 allele. J Neurosci 1997;17:516–29

Corder EH, Saunders AM, Strittmatter WJ, et al. Gene dose of apolipoprotein E type 4 allele and the risk of Alzheimer's disease in late onset families. Science 1993;261:921–3

Farrer LA, Cupples LA, Haines JL, et al. Effects of age, sex and ethnicity on the association between apolipoprotein E genotype and Alzheimer disease. A meta-analysis. J Am Med Assoc 1997;278:1349–56

Poirier J, Davignon J, Bouthillier D, et al. Apolipoprotein E polymorphism and Alzheimer's disease. Lancet 1993;342:697–9

Poirier J. Apolipoprotein E in animal models of CNS injury and in Alzheimer's disase. Trends Neurosci 1994;17:525–30

Poirier J, Delisle M-C, Quirion R, et al. Apolipoprotein E4 allele as a predictor of cholinergic deficits and treatment outcome in Alzheimer's disease. Proc Natl Acad Sci USA 1995;92:12260–4

Presenilin 1 and presenilin 2

Hutton M, Hardy J. The presenilins and Alzheimer's disease. Hum Mol Genet 1997;6:1639–46

Lendon CL, Ashall F, Goate AM. Exploring the etiology of Alzheimer's disease using molecular genetics. J Am Med Assoc 1997;277:825–31

Mattson MP, Guo Q. Cell and molecular neurobiology of presenilins: A role for the endoplasmic reticulum in the pathogenesis of Alzheimer's disease? J Neurosci Res 1997;50:505–13

Kim TW, Tanzi RE. Presenilins and Alzheimer's disease. Curr Opin Neurobiol 1997;7:683–8

Amyloid precursor protein and β-amyloid

Chartier-Harlin M-C, Crawford F, Houlden H, et al. Early-onset Alzheimer's disease caused by mutations at codon 717 of the beta amyloid precursor gene. Nature 1991;353:844–6

Goate A, Chartier-Harlin MC, Mullan M, et al. Segregation of a mis-sense mutation in the amyloid precursor protein gene with familial Alzheimer's disease. Nature 1991;349:704–6

Haass C, Koo EH, Mellon A, et al. Targeting of cell-surface beta amyloid precursor protein to lysosome: Alternative processing into amyloid-bearing fragments. Nature 1992;357:500–3

Sisodia SS, Koo EH, Beyreuther K, et al. Evidence that beta amyloid protein in Alzheimer's disease is not derived by normal processing. Science 1990;248:492–5

Yankner BA, Dawes RL, Fisher S, et al. Neurotoxicity of a fragment of the amyloid precursor protein associated with Alzheimer's disease. Science 1989;245:417–20

Index